Foot and
Ankle Anatomy

Color Atlas of
Foot and
Ankle Anatomy

R M H McMinn

Conservator of the Hunterian Museum
Formerly Sir William Collins Professor
of Human and Comparative Anatomy
Royal College of Surgeons of England

R T Hutchings

Photographer
Formerly Chief Medical Laboratory
Scientific Officer, Royal College
of Surgeons of England

B M Logan

Prosector
Department of Anatomy
Royal College of Surgeons of England

APPLETON-CENTURY-CROFTS/Connecticut

A Division of Prentice-Hall, Inc.

General Editor, Wolfe Medical Atlases:
G. Barry Carruthers, MD(Lond)

Copyright © R. M. H. McMinn, R. T. Hutchings &
B. M. Logan, 1982
Published by Wolfe Medical Publications Ltd, 1982
Printed by Royal Smeets Offset b.v.,
Weert, Netherlands

Distributed in Continental North America by
Appleton-Century-Crofts, 25 Van Zant Street,
East Norwalk, Connecticut 06855

Library of Congress Catalog Number: 82-50763
ISBN: 0-8385-1172-4

This book is one of the titles in the series of
Wolfe Medical Atlases, a series which brings
together probably the world's largest systematic
published collection of diagnostic colour
photographs.
For a full list of Atlases in the series, plus
forthcoming titles and details of our surgical,
dental and veterinary Atlases, please write to
Wolfe Medical Publications Ltd, Wolfe House,
3 Conway Street, London W1P 6HE.

Preface

This atlas provides photographic illustrations of the anatomy of the normal adult human foot. After a short introduction to some of the major features of the whole lower limb, the photographs of the foot itself are natural size, so that those who are examining the living foot or studying bones and dissections can readily correlate the specimens with the pictures and appreciate the actual sizes of different structures. A number of notes on some items have been included in order to emphasise important features or explain difficult points, but there has been no attempt to provide a comprehensive textual coverage. The atlas is intended to complement other texts, atlases and dissecting manuals, not to replace them. The system of using overlying identification numbers with an adjacent key allows students to test their knowledge by covering up the key.

The foot is of professional importance not only to medical students and practitioners and specialists groups such as orthopaedic surgeons, chiropodists, podiatrists, physiotherapists and nurses, but to others such as dancers and athletes. Those engaged in all kinds of sporting activities may be interested in information about its normal anatomy. We hope that all who use the atlas will derive instruction and pleasure from it.

R M H McMinn
R T Hutchings
B M Logan

To
Christopher and Jacqueline
Sam and Isabel
and Evelyn

Acknowledgements

For helpful discussions during the preparation of this book we are much indebted to Mr Leslie Klenerman, Consultant Orthopaedic Surgeon, Northwick Park Hospital, Harrow, and to our anatomical colleague Dr D H Bosman. We are also grateful to Mr W Stripp, Superintendent Radiographer at the Royal National Orthopaedic Hospital, Great Portland Street, London, for providing the radiographs, and to Gina Howes for the typing of the manuscript.

Contents

The Lower Limb   10–17

   Bones, muscles and surface landmarks of the left lower
     limb,
     from the front   10
     from behind   12
     from the medial side   14
     from the lateral side   16

The Leg and Foot   18–19

   Muscles of the left leg and foot   18

Surface Landmarks of the Foot   20–23

   Surface landmarks of the left foot,
     from the front and behind   20
     from below   21
     from the medial side   22
     from the lateral side   23

Skeleton of the Foot   24–33

   The disarticulated bones of the left foot,
     from above   24
   The articulated bones of the left foot,
     from above and below   26
   Attachments of muscles and major ligaments to the
     bones of the left foot   28
   The articulated bones of the left foot,
     from the medial and lateral sides   30
   The bones of the left longitudinal arches,
     the transverse tarsal joint, and other joints   32

Individual Foot Bones   34–49

   The left talus   34
   The left talus with the lower ends of the tibia and fibula   36
   The left talus with the lower ends of the tibia and fibula,
     with ligamentous attachments   38
   The left talus with the lower ends of the tibia and fibula   40
   The left talus with the lower ends of the tibia and fibula,
     with ligamentous attachments   42
   The left calcaneus   44
   The left navicular and cuboid bones   46
   The left cuneiform bones   47
   The left metatarsal bones   48

Dissection of the Dorsum and Sides of the Foot   50–62

   Superficial vessels and nerves of the left foot,
     from the front   50
     from behind   51
     from the medial side   52
     from the lateral side   53

   The deep fascia of the right foot,
     from the front and the right   54

   Muscles, nerves and vessels of the right foot,
     from the front   56
     from behind   57
     from the medial side   58
     from the lateral side   59

   Deep nerves and vessels of the dorsum of the left foot   60
   The left foot from above with the talus removed   62

Dissection of the Sole of the Foot   63–67

  The left plantar aponeurosis and cutaneous nerves   63
  The left sole: the first layer of muscles   64
  The left sole: the second layer of muscles   65
  The left sole: the third layer of muscles   66
  The left sole: the fourth layer of muscles   67

Ligaments of the Foot   68–71

  Ligaments of the right foot,
    from above, the lateral side and behind   69
    from the medial side   70
    ligaments of the sole   71

Sections of the Foot   72–83

  Sagittal sections of the right foot,
    through the great toe   72
    through the second toe   74
    through the fifth toe   75
  Sections of the right lower leg and foot, above, through
    and below the ankle joint   76
  Coronal sections of the left ankle joint   78
  Oblique horizontal sections of the left foot   80
  Sections of the right tarsus   82
  Sections of the right metatarsus   83

The Great Toe   84

  The dorsum, nail, and sections of the great toe   84

Radiography of the Foot   85–87

Anteroposterior and lateral radiographs   85
Miscellaneous radiographs   86

Appendix   88
  Muscles   88
  Nerves   92
  Arteries   92

Index   94

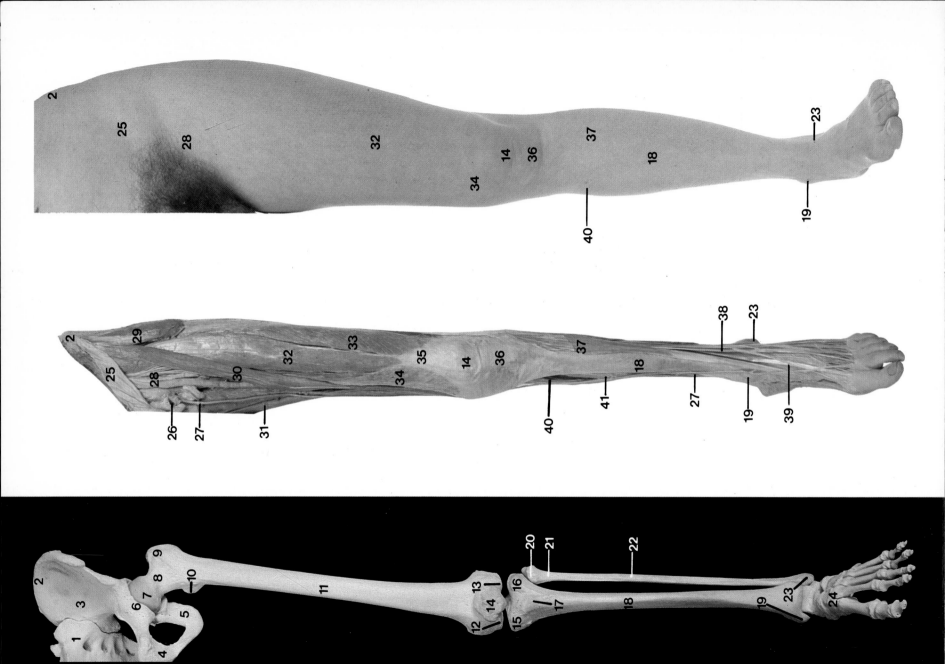

The lower limb

Bones, muscles and surface landmarks of the left lower limb, from the front

1 Sacrum
2 Iliac crest
3 Ilium ⎤
4 Pubis ⎬ hip bone
5 Ischium ⎦
6 Rim of acetabulum
7 Head ⎤
8 Neck ⎥
9 Greater trochanter ⎬ of femur
10 Lesser trochanter ⎥
11 Body (shaft) ⎦
12 Medial condyle
13 Lateral condyle
14 Patella
15 Medial condyle ⎤
16 Lateral condyle ⎥
17 Tuberosity ⎬ of tibia
18 Body (shaft) ⎥
19 Medial malleolus ⎦
20 Head ⎤
21 Neck ⎬ of fibula
22 Body (shaft) ⎥
23 Lateral malleolus ⎦
24 Foot
25 Inguinal ligament
26 Inguinal lymph nodes
27 Great saphenous vein
28 Femoral triangle, vessels and nerve
29 Tensor fasciae latae
30 Sartorius
31 Gracilis
32 Rectus femoris
33 Vastus lateralis
34 Vastus medialis
35 Quadriceps tendon
36 Patellar ligament
37 Tibialis anterior
38 Extensor digitorum longus
39 Extensor hallucis longus
40 Gastrocnemius
41 Soleus

- The main parts or regions of the lower limb are the gluteal region (consisting of the hip at the side and the buttock at the back), the thigh, the knee, the leg, the ankle and the foot. The term leg properly refers to the part between the knee and the foot, although it is commonly used for the whole lower limb.

- The hip bone consists of three bones fused together – the ilium, ischium and pubis – and forms a pelvic girdle. The two hip bones or girdles unite with each other in front at the pubic symphysis, and at the back they join the sacrum at the sacro-iliac joints, so forming the bony pelvis.

- The femur is the bone of the thigh; the tibia and fibula are the bones of the leg.

- The acetabulum of the hip bone and the head of the femur form the hip joint.

- The condyles of the femur and tibia together with the patella form the knee joint.

- The head of the fibula forms a small joint with the tibia, the superior tibiofibular joint. The inferior tibiofibular joint is a fibrous union between the tibia and fibula just above the ankle joint.

- The ankle is the lower part of the leg in the region of the ankle joint.

- The lower ends of the tibia and fibula articulate with the talus of the foot to form the ankle joint.

- The body of a long bone is commonly called the shaft.

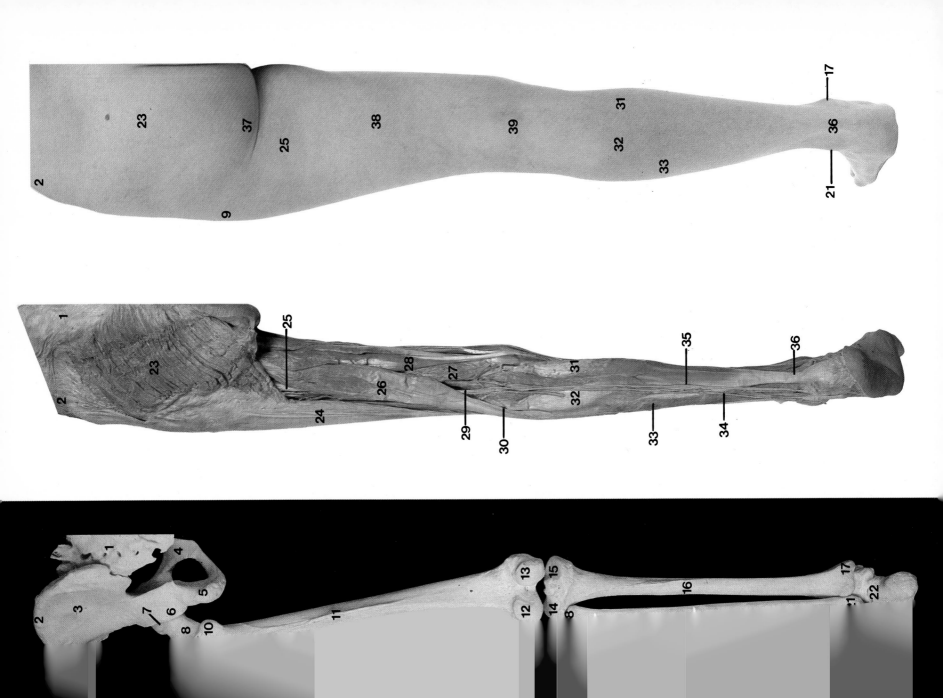

The lower limb

Bones, muscles and surface landmarks of the left lower limb, from behind

1 Sacrum
2 Iliac crest
3 Ilium
4 Pubis
5 Ischium
6 Rim of acetabulum
7 Head
8 Neck
9 Greater trochanter
10 Lesser trochanter
11 Body
12 Medial condyle
13 Lateral condyle
14 Medial condyle
15 Lateral condyle
16 Body
17 Medial malleolus
18 Head
19 Neck
20 Body
21 Lateral malleolus
22 Foot
23 Gluteus maximus
24 Iliotibial tract
25 Sciatic nerve
26 Biceps femoris
27 Semimembranosus
28 Semitendinosus
29 Tibial nerve
30 Common peroneal nerve
31 Medial head
32 Lateral head
33 Soleus
34 Sural nerve
35 Small saphenous vein
36 Tendo calcaneus
37 Fold of buttock
38 Hamstring muscles
39 Popliteal fossa

of femur

of tibia

of fibula

of gastrocnemius

● The tendons of gastrocnemius and soleus join to form the tendo calcaneus, commonly known as the Achilles tendon.

● The muscles on the back of the thigh with prominent tendons – semimembranosus, semitendinosus and biceps (long head) – are commonly known as the hamstrings.

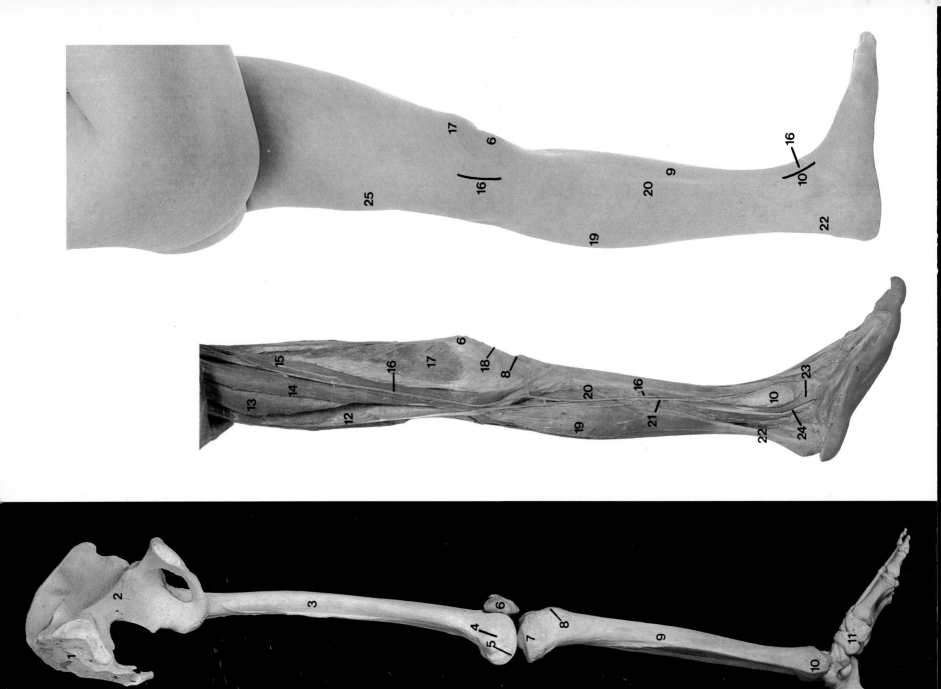

The lower limb

Bones, muscles and surface landmarks of the left lower limb, from the medial side

1 Sacrum
2 Hip bone
3 Body
4 Medial epicondyle
5 Medial condyle ⎤ of femur
6 Patella
7 Medial condyle
8 Tuberosity ⎤ of tibia
9 Body
10 Medial malleolus
11 Foot
12 Semitendinosus
13 Semimembranosus
14 Gracilis
15 Sartorius
16 Great saphenous vein
17 Vastus medialis
18 Patellar ligament
19 Gastrocnemius
20 Soleus
21 Saphenous nerve
22 Tendo calcaneus
23 Tibialis posterior
24 Flexor digitorum longus
25 Hamstrings

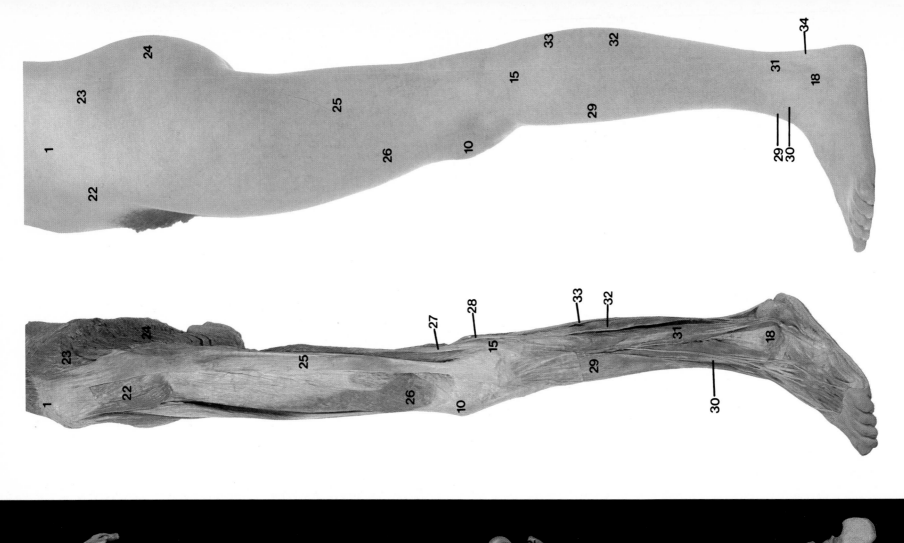
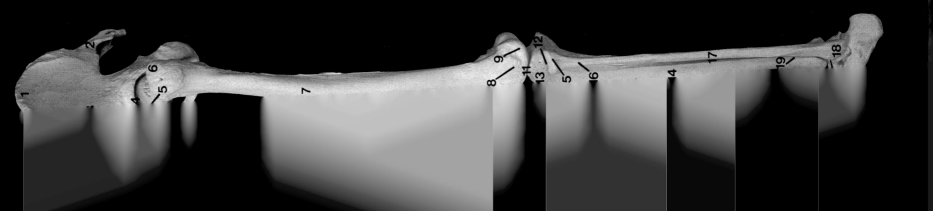

The lower limb

Bones, muscles and surface landmarks of the left lower limb, from the lateral side

1 Iliac crest
2 Sacrum
3 Hip bone
4 Hip joint
5 Head ⎱
6 Greater trochanter
7 Body ⎰ of femur
8 Lateral epicondyle
9 Lateral condyle
10 Patella
11 Knee joint
12 Superior tibiofibular joint
13 Lateral condyle ⎱ of tibia
14 Body ⎰
15 Head ⎱
16 Neck of fibula
17 Body ⎰
18 Lateral malleolus
19 Inferior tibiofibular joint
20 Ankle joint
21 Foot
22 Tensor fasciae latae
23 Gluteus medius
24 Gluteus maximus
25 Iliotibial tract
26 Vastus lateralis
27 Biceps femoris
28 Common peroneal nerve
29 Tibialis anterior
30 Extensor digitorum longus
31 Peroneus longus
32 Soleus
33 Gastrocnemius
34 Tendo calcaneus

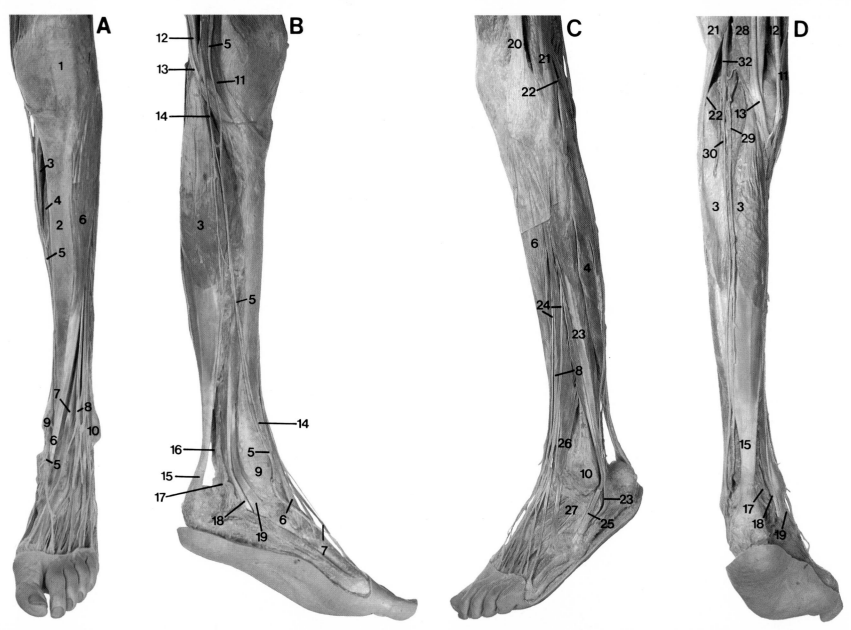

The leg and foot

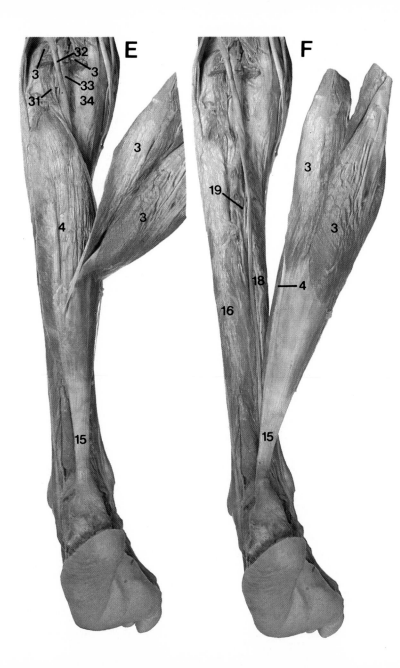

Muscles of the left leg and foot (after removal of most of the deep fascia)

A From the front
B From the medial side
C From the lateral side
D From behind
E From behind with gastrocnemius removed and reflected medially

F From behind with plantaris, gastrocnemius and soleus removed and reflected medially

 1 Patellar ligament
 2 Medial surface of tibia
 3 Gastrocnemius
 4 Soleus
 5 Great saphenous vein
 6 Tibialis anterior
 7 Extensor hallucis longus
 8 Extensor digitorum longus
 9 Medial malleolus
10 Lateral malleolus
11 Sartorius
12 Gracilis
13 Semitendinosus
14 Saphenous nerve
15 Tendo calcaneus
16 Flexor hallucis longus
17 Tibial nerve and posterior tibial vessels
18 Flexor digitorum longus
19 Tibialis posterior
20 Iliotibial tract
21 Biceps femoris
22 Common peroneal nerve
23 Peroneus longus
24 Superficial peroneal nerve
25 Peroneus brevis
26 Peroneus tertius
27 Externsor digitorum brevis
28 Semimembranosus
29 Small saphenous vein
30 Sural nerve
31 Plantaris
32 Tibial nerve
33 Popliteal vein overlying artery
34 Fascia over popliteus

● **Muscles of the leg and foot**

 Extensor muscles of the front of the leg and dorsum of the foot
  Tibialis anterior
  Extensor hallucis longus
  Extensor digitorum longus
  Peroneus tertius
  Extensor digitorum brevis
 Peroneal muscles of the lateral side of the leg
  Peroneus longus
  Peroneus brevis
 Flexor muscles of the back of the leg and sole of the foot
  Gastrocnemius
  Soleus
  Plantaris
  Popliteus
  Tibialis posterior
  Flexor hallucis longus
  Flexor digitorum longus
 Muscles of the sole – see page 64.

For a summary of muscles and attachments, nerve supplies and actions see page 88.

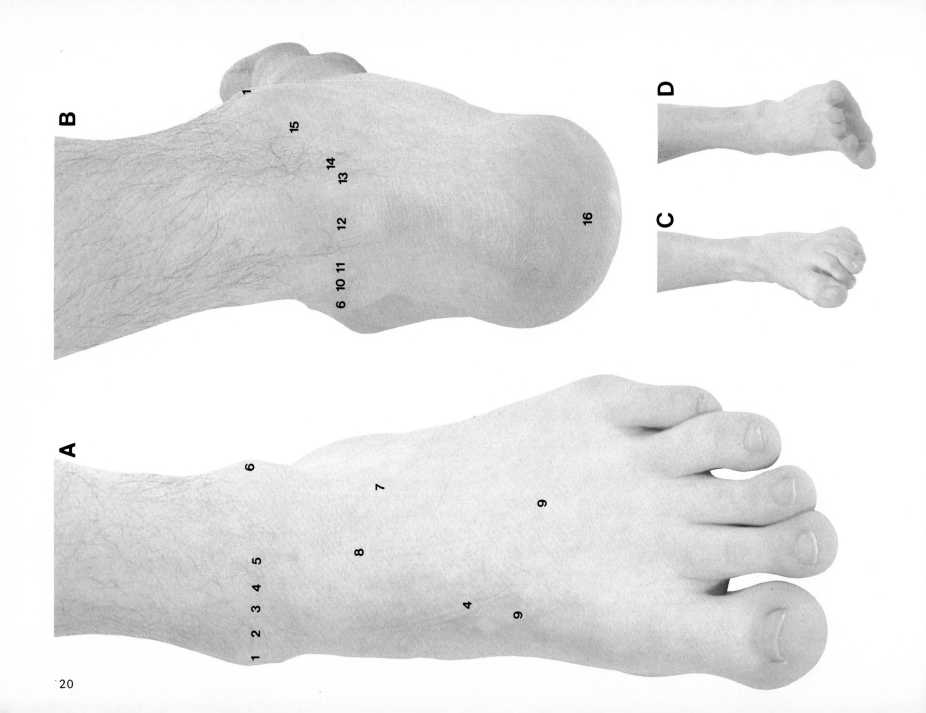

20

Surface landmarks of the foot

Surface landmarks of the left foot

A From the front (dorsal surface, dorsum)
B From behind
C From the front, in inversion
D From the front, in eversion with abduction of toes
E From below (plantar surface, sole)
F Imprint of sole when weight-bearing

1 Medial malleolus
2 Great saphenous vein and saphenous nerve
3 Tibialis anterior
4 Extensor hallucis longus
5 Extensor digitorum longus
6 Lateral malleolus
7 Extensor digitorum brevis
8 Dorsalis pedis artery
9 Dorsal venous arch
10 Peroneus longus and brevis
11 Small saphenous vein and sural nerve
12 Tendo calcaneus
13 Flexor hallucis longus
14 Posterior tibial artery and tibial nerve
15 Flexor digitorum longus and tibialis posterior
16 Tuberosity of calcaneus
17 Sesamoid bones under head of first metatarsal
18 Base of first metatarsal
19 Head of fifth metatarsal
20 Tuberosity of base of fifth metatarsal
21 Tuberosity of navicular

● **Definition of movements**

Extension: from the Latin for straightening out, but as far as the ankle and foot are concerned it means bending the foot or toes upwards, and is also known as dorsiflexion.

Flexion: from the Latin for bending. In the ankle and foot it means bending the foot or toes downwards, which is also known as plantar flexion.

Abduction: from the Latin for moving away. In the foot it means spreading the toes apart (the corresponding movement of the fingers is much more extensive).

Adduction: from the Latin for moving towards. In the foot it means drawing the toes together.

Inversion: from the Latin for turning in – turning the foot so that the sole faces more inwards (medially).

Eversion: from the Latin for turning out – moving the foot so that the sole faces more outwards (laterally) (a more limited movement than inversion).

For further details see pages 67 and 79.

E

F

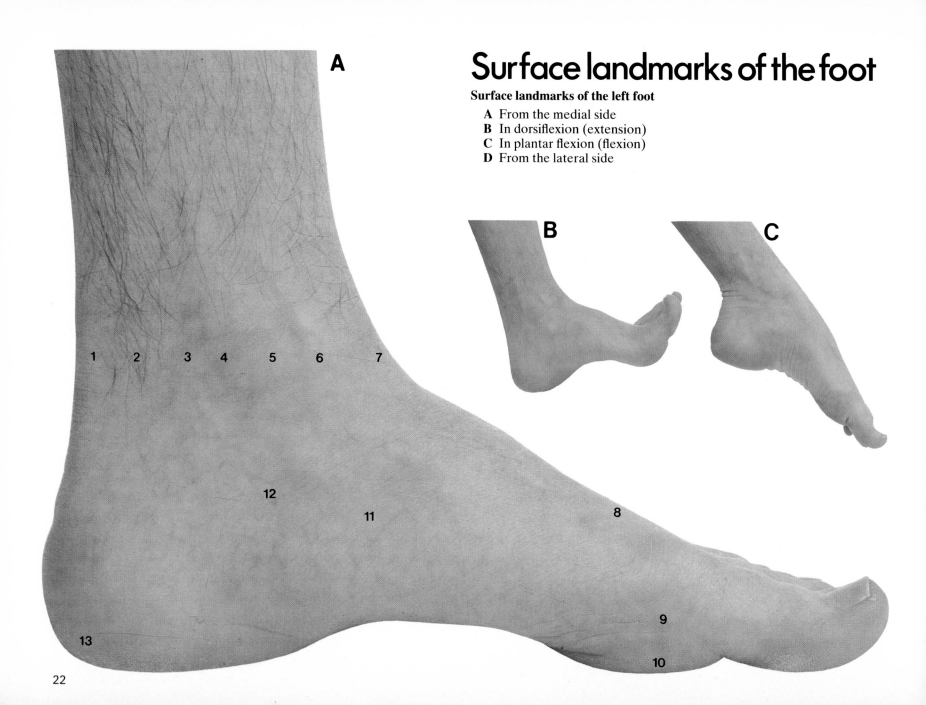

Surface landmarks of the foot

Surface landmarks of the left foot

A From the medial side
B In dorsiflexion (extension)
C In plantar flexion (flexion)
D From the lateral side

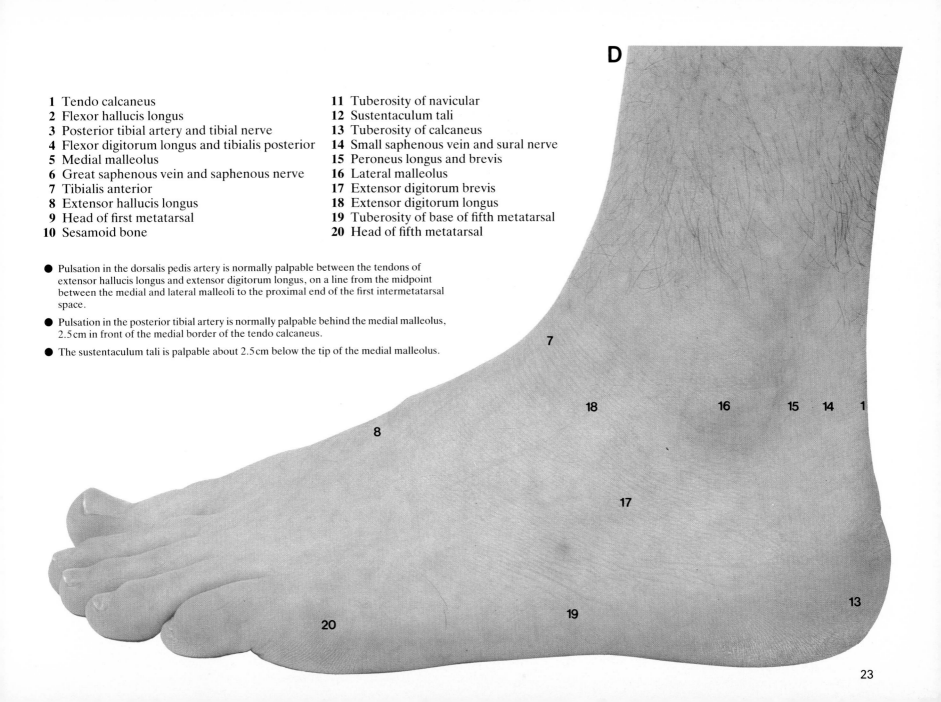

D

1 Tendo calcaneus
2 Flexor hallucis longus
3 Posterior tibial artery and tibial nerve
4 Flexor digitorum longus and tibialis posterior
5 Medial malleolus
6 Great saphenous vein and saphenous nerve
7 Tibialis anterior
8 Extensor hallucis longus
9 Head of first metatarsal
10 Sesamoid bone

11 Tuberosity of navicular
12 Sustentaculum tali
13 Tuberosity of calcaneus
14 Small saphenous vein and sural nerve
15 Peroneus longus and brevis
16 Lateral malleolus
17 Extensor digitorum brevis
18 Extensor digitorum longus
19 Tuberosity of base of fifth metatarsal
20 Head of fifth metatarsal

● Pulsation in the dorsalis pedis artery is normally palpable between the tendons of extensor hallucis longus and extensor digitorum longus, on a line from the midpoint between the medial and lateral malleoli to the proximal end of the first intermetatarsal space.

● Pulsation in the posterior tibial artery is normally palpable behind the medial malleolus, 2.5 cm in front of the medial border of the tendo calcaneus.

● The sustentaculum tali is palpable about 2.5 cm below the tip of the medial malleolus.

23

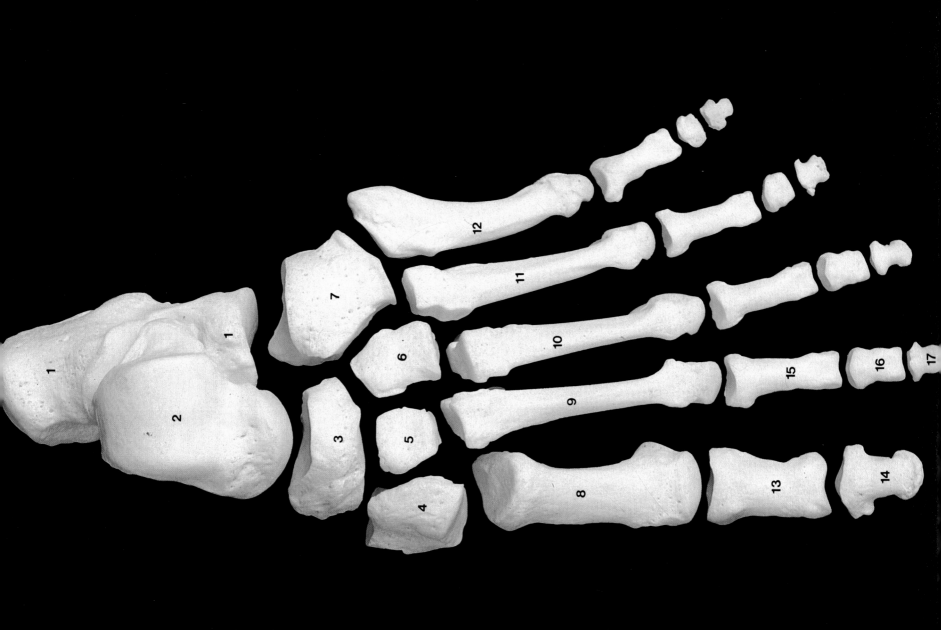

Skeleton of the foot

The disarticulated bones of the left foot, from above

(The talus and calcaneus remain articulated)

1 Calcaneus
2 Talus
3 Navicular
4 Medial cuneiform
5 Intermediate cuneiform
6 Lateral cuneiform
7 Cuboid
8 First metatarsal
9 Second metatarsal
10 Third metatarsal
11 Fourth metatarsal
12 Fifth metatarsal
13 Proximal phalanx of great toe
14 Distal phalanx of great toe
15 Proximal phalanx of second toe
16 Middle phalanx of second toe
17 Distal phalanx of second toe

● **Bones of the tarsus, the back part of the foot**
  Talus
  Calcaneus
  Navicular bone
  Cuboid bone
  Medial, intermediate and lateral cuneiform bones

● **Bones of the metatarsus, the forepart of the foot**
  First to fifth metatarsal bones (numbered from the medial side)

● **Bones of the toes or digits**
  Phalanges – a proximal and a distal phalanx for the great toe; proximal, middle and distal phalanges for the second to fifth toes

● **Sesamoid bones** – two always present in the tendons of flexor hallucis brevis

● **Origin and meaning of some terms associated with the foot**
  Tibia: Latin for a flute or pipe; the shin bone has a fanciful resemblance to this wind instrument.
  Fibula: Latin for a pin or skewer; the long thin bone of the leg. Adjective fibular or peroneal, which is from the Greek for pin.
  Tarsus: Greek for a wicker frame; the basic framework for the back of the foot.
  Metatarsus: Greek for beyond the tarsus; the forepart of the foot.
  Talus (astragalus): Latin (Greek) for one of a set of dice; viewed from above the main part of the talus has a rather square appearance.
  Calcaneus: from the Greek for heel; the heel bone.
  Navicular (scaphoid): Latin (Greek) for boat-shaped; the navicular bone roughly resembles a saucer-shaped coracle.
  Cuboid: Greek for cube-shaped.
  Cuneiform: Latin for wedge-shaped.
  Phalanx: Greek for a row of soldiers; a row of bones in the toes. Plural phalanges.
  Sesamoid: Greek for shaped like a sesame seed.
  Digitus: Latin for finger or toe. Digiti and digitorum are the genitive singular and genitive plural – of the toe(s).
  Hallux: Latin for the great toe. Hallucis is the genitive singular – of the great toe.
  Dorsum: Latin for back; the upper surface of the foot. Adjective dorsal.
  Plantar: adjective from planta, Latin for the sole of the foot.

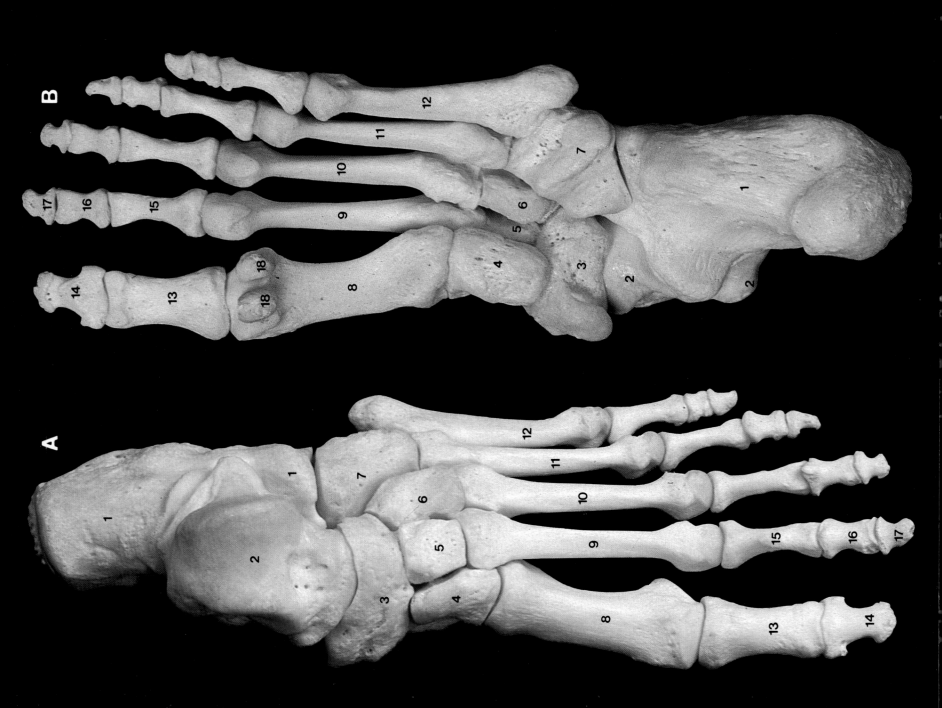

Skeleton of the foot

The articulated bones of the left foot

A From above (dorsal surface)
B From below (plantar surface)

1 Calcaneus
2 Talus
3 Navicular
4 Medial cuneiform
5 Intermediate cuneiform
6 Lateral cuneiform
7 Cuboid
8 First metatarsal
9 Second metatarsal
10 Third metatarsal
11 Fourth metatarsal
12 Fifth metatarsal
13 Proximal phalanx of great toe
14 Distal phalanx of great toe
15 Proximal phalanx of second toe
16 Middle phalanx of second toe
17 Distal phalanx of second toe
18 Sesamoid bones

Talus

The uppermost foot bone, forming the ankle joint with the tibia and fibula.

Formerly known as the astragalus.

Articular facets on the upper surface and sides for the tibia and fibula, on the under surface for the calcaneus, and on the anterior surface (head) for the navicular.

Unique among the foot bones in having no muscles attached to it.

For details see pages 34–43.

Calcaneus

The largest foot bone, forming the heel.

Formerly known as the calcaneum or os calcis.

Articular facets on the upper surface for the talus and on the anterior surface for the cuboid.

Prominent sustentaculum tali projecting medially.

For details see pages 44–45.

Navicular bone

Formerly known as the scaphoid bone.

Posterior articular facet for the talus; anterior articular facet for the three cuneiforms.

For details see page 46.

Cuboid bone

Posterior articular facet for the calcaneus; anterior articular facet for the fourth and fifth metatarsals.

Groove on the under surface for the tendon of peroneus longus.

For details see page 46.

Cuneiform bones

Medial (the largest), intermediate (the smallest), and lateral.

Situated between the navicular and the first three metatarsals.

For details see page 47.

Metatarsal bones

First to fifth, leading to each toe and each with a base (at the proximal or ankle end), body or shaft, and head (at the toe end).

Bases of first three articulate with cuneiform bones; bases of fourth and fifth articulate with the cuboid.

Heads articulate with bases of proximal phalanges.

For details see pages 48–49.

Phalanges

The bones of the toes, two for the great toe and three for the others.

Each phalanx has a base (at the proximal end), body, and head (at the distal end).

Body convex on the dorsal (upper) surface and concave on the plantar surface.

Sesamoid bones

One in each of the two tendons of flexor hallucis brevis, articulating with the plantar surface of the head of the first metatarsal.

Others may be present in similar positions in flexor tendons under other metatarsophalangeal or interphalangeal joints, or in other tendons especially those of peroneus longus and tibialis anterior.

● During the preparation of dried bones, the hyaline cartilage on articulating surfaces is lost, so that when rearticulating bones an exact fit is not possible. The thickness of the cartilage on joint surfaces is best appreciated in sections of bones, as on pages 72–83.

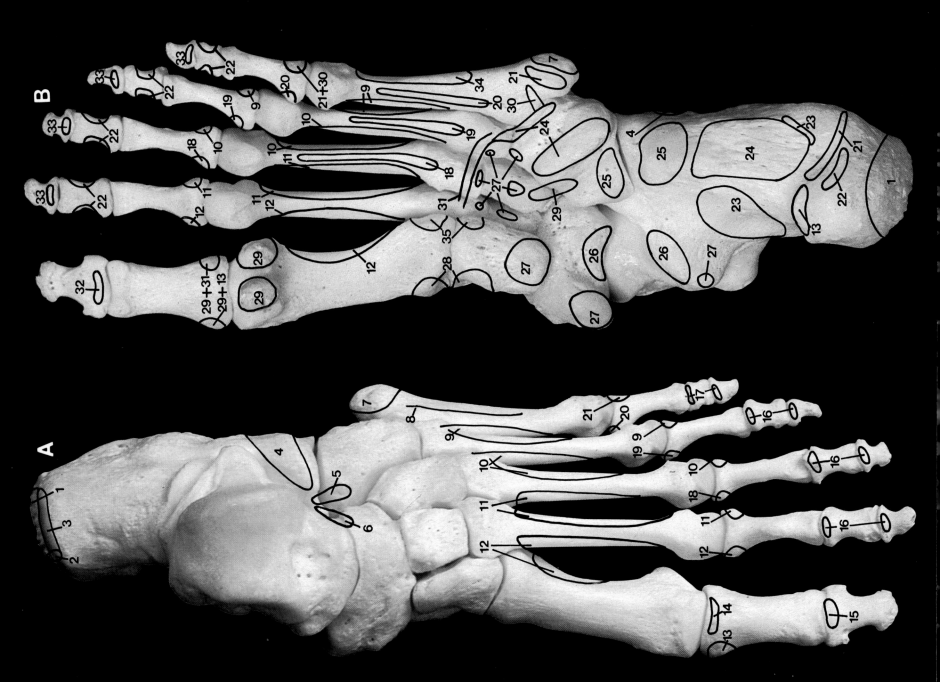

Skeleton of the foot

Attachments of muscles and major ligaments to the bones of the left foot

A From above (dorsal surface)
B From below (plantar surface)

1 Tendo calcaneus
2 Plantaris
3 Area for bursa
4 Extensor digitorum brevis
5 Calcaneocuboid part of bifurcate ligament
6 Calcaneonavicular part of bifurcate ligament
7 Peroneus brevis
8 Peroneus tertius
9 Fourth ⎤
10 Third ⎥ dorsal interosseous
11 Second ⎥
12 First ⎦
13 Abductor hallucis
14 Extensor hallucis brevis
15 Extensor hallucis longus
16 Extensor digitorum longus and brevis
17 Extensor digitorum longus
18 First ⎤
19 Second ⎥ plantar interosseous
20 Third ⎦
21 Abductor digiti minimi
22 Flexor digitorum brevis
23 Flexor accessorius
24 Long plantar ligament
25 Plantar calcaneocuboid (short plantar) ligament
26 Plantar calcaneonavicular (spring) ligament
27 Tibialis posterior
28 Tibialis anterior
29 Flexor hallucis brevis
30 Flexor digiti minimi brevis
31 Adductor hallucis
32 Flexor hallucis longus
33 Flexor digitorum longus
34 Opponens digiti minimi (occasional part of 30)
35 Peroneus longus

● Flexor accessorius is alternatively known as quadratus plantae.

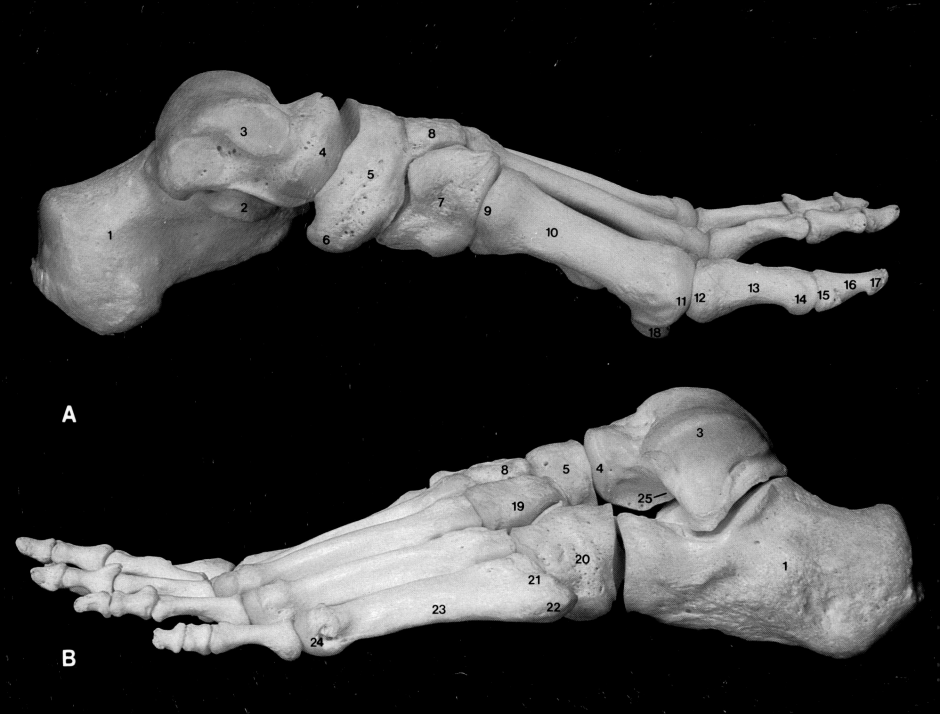

A

B

Skeleton of the foot

The articulated bones of the left foot

  A From the medial side
  B From the lateral side

  1 Calcaneus
  2 Sustentaculum tali
  3 Talus
  4 Head of talus
  5 Navicular
  6 Tuberosity of navicular
  7 Medial cuneiform
  8 Intermediate cuneiform
  9 Base ⎤
10 Body ⎬ of first metatarsal
11 Head ⎦
12 Base ⎤
13 Body ⎬ of proximal phalanx of great toe
14 Head ⎦
15 Base ⎤
16 Body ⎬ of distal phalanx of great toe
17 Head ⎦
18 Sesamoid bone
19 Lateral cuneiform
20 Cuboid
21 Base ⎤
22 Tuberosity ⎬ of fifth metatarsal
23 Body ⎪
24 Head ⎦
25 Tarsal sinus

● When standing (as can be seen from the imprint of a wet foot on the floor – page 21) the parts of the foot in contact with the ground are the heel, the lateral margin of the foot, the pads under the metatarsal heads and the pads under the distal part of the toes.

● The medial margin of the foot is not normally in contact with the ground because of the height of the medial longitudinal arch. In flat foot the medial arch is lower with an increasingly large imprint on the medial side.

● The body weight when standing is borne by the tuberosity of the calcaneus and the heads of the metatarsals, especially the first (with the sesamoid bones underneath it) and the fifth. As the foot bends forwards in walking the other metatarsal heads take increasingly more of the load. With further raising of the heel the toe pads become pressed to the ground and so take some of the weight off the metatarsals.

● Although the forearm and hand have many muscles that are similar in name and action to those of the leg and foot, their normal use in everyday life is different.

In the upper limb the muscles work from above to produce intricate movements of the thumb and fingers in a free limb.

In the lower limb the toes have to be stabilised on the ground so that muscles can work from below to produce the propulsive movements of walking.

- The bones of the medial longitudinal arch are the calcaneus, talus, navicular, three cuneiforms and the medial three metatarsal bones.

- The bones of the lateral longitudinal arch are the calcaneus, the cuboid and the two lateral metatarsal bones.

- The transverse arch is formed by the cuboid and cuneiform bones and the adjacent parts of the five metatarsals (those of each foot forming one half of the whole arch). At the level of the metatarsal heads the arched form is no longer present.

- The medial longitudinal arch is higher than the lateral.

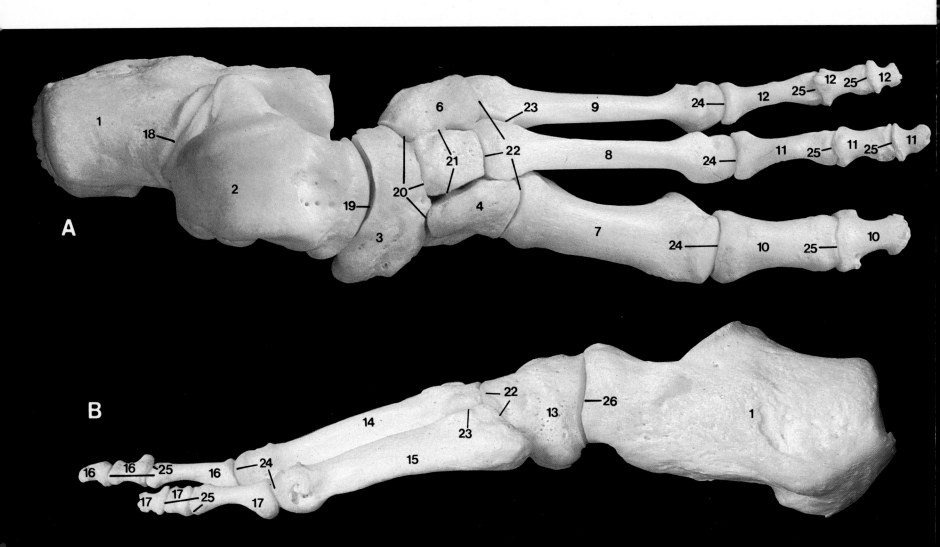

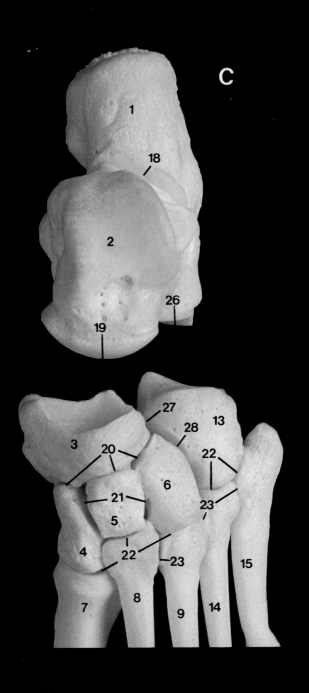

- While the shape of the individual bones determines the shape of the arches, the *maintenance* of the arches in the *stationary* foot (standing in the normal upright position) depends largely on the ligaments in the sole (where they are larger and stronger than those on the dorsum). As soon as movement occurs the long tendons and small muscles of the sole assume importance in maintaining the curved forms.

- The many joints of the foot contribute to its function as a *flexible* lever, and the word arch suggests an architectural rigidity that does not exist.

- On the medial side the plantar calcaneonavicular ligament (spring ligament) is of particular importance in supporting the head of the talus, and other structures that help to maintain the medial arch include the plantar aponeurosis, flexor hallucis longus, tibialis anterior and posterior, and the medial parts of flexor digitorum longus and brevis.

- In maintaining the lateral arch, particular importance is attached to peroneus longus, the plantar aponeurosis, the long plantar ligament, the plantar calcaneocuboid (short plantar) ligament, and the lateral parts of flexor digitorum longus and brevis.

- The transverse tarsal joint (midtarsal joint) is the collective name for two joints – the calcaneocuboid joint, and the talonavicular part of the talocalcaneonavicular joint.

Skeleton of the foot

The bones of the left longitudinal arches, the transverse tarsal joint, and other joints

    A Bones of the medial longitudinal arch, from above
    B Bones of the lateral longitudinal arch, from the lateral side
    C The transverse tarsal joint, disarticulated, from above

1 Calcaneus	**12** Phalanges of third toe	**22** Tarsometatarsal joints
2 Talus	**13** Cuboid	(cuneometatarsal and
3 Navicular	**14** Fourth metatarsal	cuboideometatarsal)
4 Medial cuneiform	**15** Fifth metatarsal	**23** Intermetatarsal joints
5 Intermediate cuneiform	**16** Phalanges of fourth toe	**24** Metatarsophalangeal joints
6 Lateral cuneiform	**17** Phalanges of fifth toe	**25** Interphalangeal joints
7 First metatarsal	**18** Talocalcanean joint	**26** Calcaneocuboid joint
8 Second metatarsal	**19** Talonavicular part of	**27** Cuboideonavicular joint
9 Third metatarsal	talocalcaneonavicular joint	**28** Cuneocuboid joint
10 Phalanges of great toe	**20** Cuneonavicular joint	
11 Phalanges of second toe	**21** Intercuneiform joints	

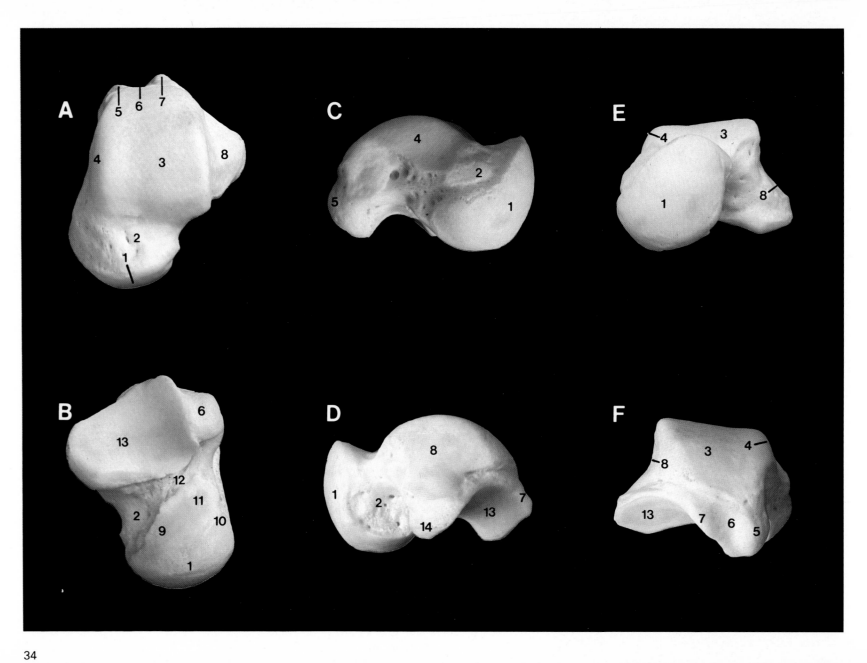

34

Individual foot bones

The left talus

- **A** From above
- **B** From below
- **C** From the medial side
- **D** From the lateral side
- **E** From the front
- **F** From behind

- **1** Head with articular surface for navicular
- **2** Neck
- **3** Trochlear surface of body, for inferior surface of tibia
- **4** Surface for medial malleolus
- **5** Medial tubercle
- **6** Groove for flexor hallucis longus tendon ⎤ of posterior process
- **7** Lateral tubercle ⎦
- **8** Surface for lateral malleolus
- **9** Anterior calcanean articular surface
- **10** Surface for plantar calcaneonavicular (spring) ligament
- **11** Middle calcanean articular surface
- **12** Sulcus tali
- **13** Posterior calcanean articular surface
- **14** Lateral process

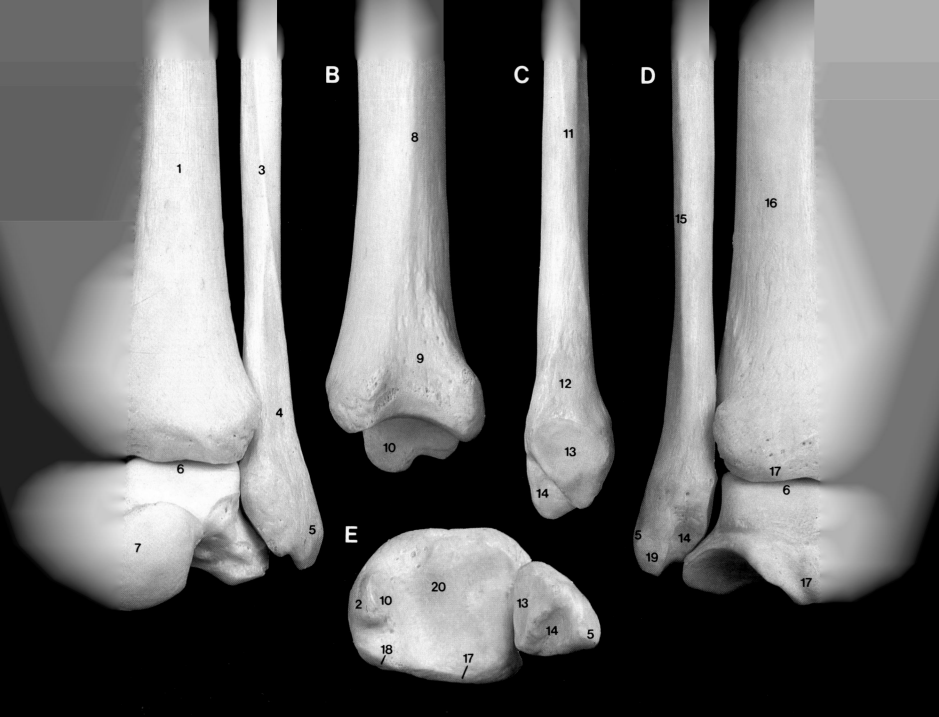

Individual foot bones

The left talus with the lower ends of the tibia and fibula

  A The talus, tibia and fibula, articulated, from the front
  B The tibia from the lateral side
  C The fibula from the medial side
  D The talus, tibia and fibula, articulated, from behind
  E The tibia and fibula, articulated, from below

  1 Anterior surface ⎤
  2 Medial malleolus ⎦ of tibia
  3 Anterior border ⎤
  4 Triangular subcutaneous area ⎬ of fibula
  5 Lateral malleolus ⎦
  6 Trochlear surface of body ⎤
  7 Head ⎦ of talus
  8 Interosseous border ⎤
  9 Fibular notch ⎬ of tibia
 10 Articular (lateral) surface of medial malleolus ⎦
 11 Interosseous border ⎤
 12 Surface for interosseous tibiofibular ligament ⎟
 13 Articular (medial) surface of lateral malleolus ⎬ of fibula
 14 Malleolar fossa ⎟
 15 Posterior border ⎦
 16 Posterior surface of tibia
 17 Groove for flexor hallucis longus
 18 Groove for tibialis posterior
 19 Groove for peroneus brevis
 20 Inferior surface of tibia

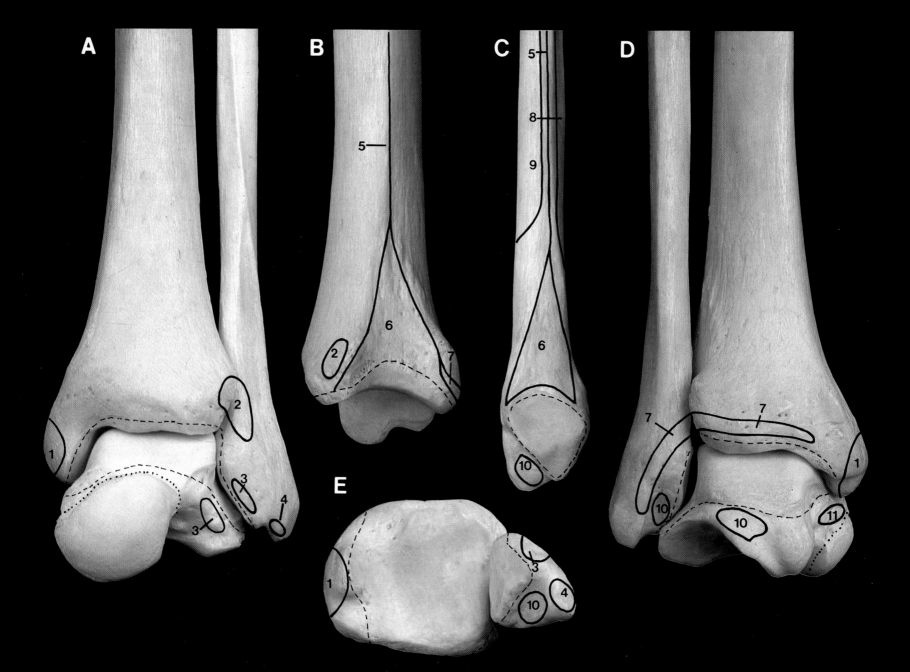

Individual foot bones

The left talus with the lower ends of the tibia and fibula, showing ligamentous attachments in the ankle region

(The attachment of the capsule of the ankle joint is indicated by the interrupted line, and that of the talocalcaneonavicular joint by the dotted line.)

A The talus, tibia and fibula, articulated, from the front
B The tibia from the lateral side
C The fibula from the medial side
D The talus, tibia and fibula, articulated, from behind
E The tibia and fibula, articulated, from below

1 Medial (deltoid) ligament
2 Anterior tibiofibular ligament
3 Anterior talofibular ligament
4 Calcaneofibular ligament
5 Interosseous membrane
6 Interosseous tibiofibular ligament
7 Posterior tibiofibular ligament
8 Peroneus tertius
9 Flexor hallucis longus
10 Posterior talofibular ligament
11 Deep part of medial (deltoid) ligament

For illustrations of ligaments and joints see pages 68–71.

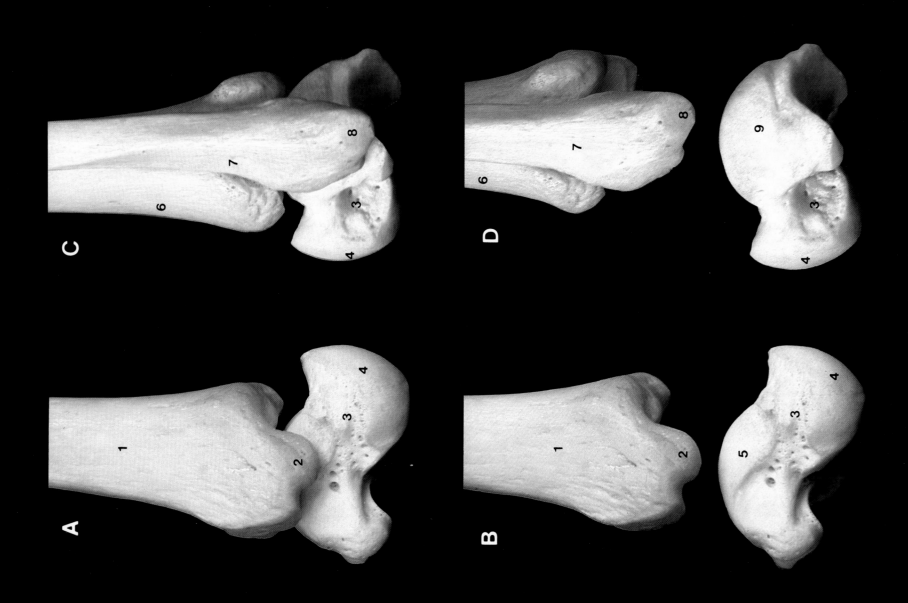

Individual foot bones

The left talus with the lower ends of the tibia and fibula

A The talus and tibia, articulated, from the medial side

B The talus and tibia, disarticulated, from the medial side

C The talus, tibia and fibula, articulated, from the lateral side

D The talus disarticulated from the tibia and fibula, from the lateral side

1 Medial surface ⎤
2 Medial malleolus ⎦ of tibia
3 Neck ⎤
4 Head ⎦ of talus
5 Surface for medial malleolus
6 Anterior surface of tibia
7 Triangular subcutaneous surface ⎤
8 Lateral malleolus ⎦ of fibula
9 Surface for lateral malleolus

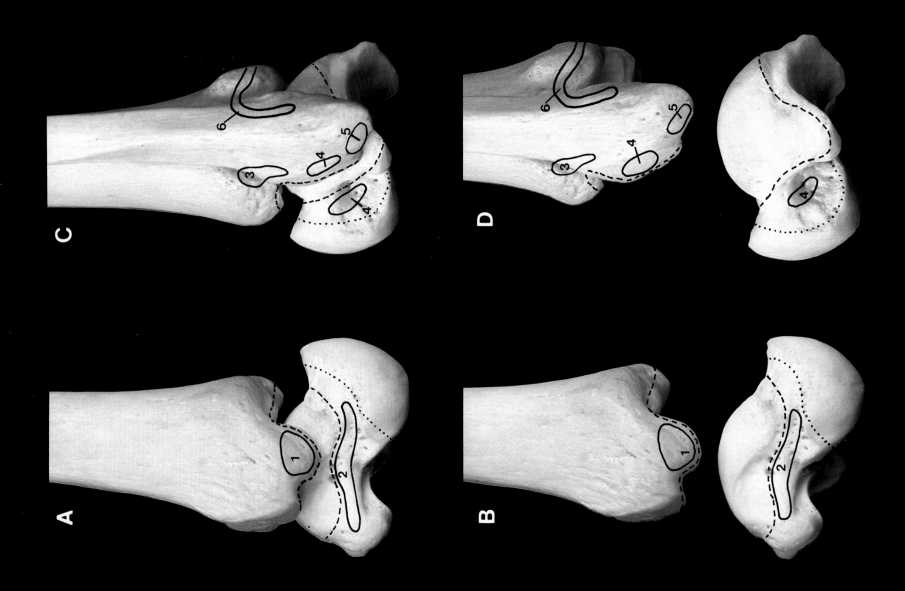

Individual foot bones

The left talus with the lower ends of the tibia and fibula, showing ligamentous attachments in the ankle region

(The attachment of the capsule of the ankle joint is indicated by the interrupted line, and that of the talocalcaneonavicular joint by the dotted line)

A The talus and tibia, articulated, from the medial side

B The talus and tibia, disarticulated, from the medial side

C The talus, tibia and fibula, articulated, from the lateral side

D The talus, disarticulated from the tibia and fibula, from the lateral side

1 Medial (deltoid) ligament
2 Deep part of medial (deltoid) ligament
3 Anterior tibiofibular ligament
4 Anterior talofibular ligament
5 Calcaneofibular ligament
6 Posterior tibiofibular ligament

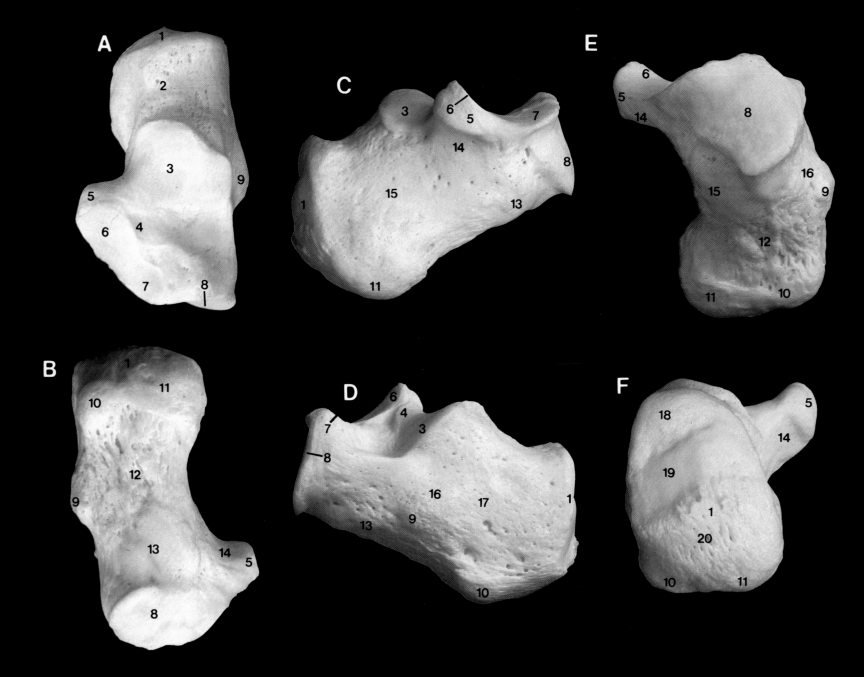

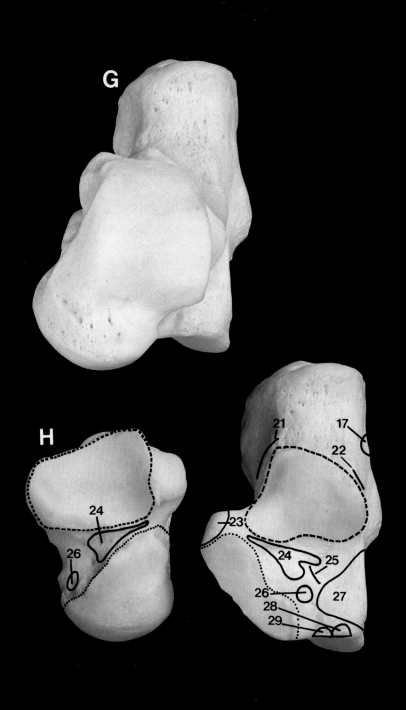

Individual foot bones

The left calcaneus

A From above
B From below
C From the medial side
D From the lateral side
E From the front
F From behind
G Articulated with the talus, from above

H With the talus disarticulated and turned upside down, with attachments
(Capsule of talocalcanean joint: interrupted line. Capsule of talocalcanean part of talocalcaneonavicular joint: dotted line)

 1 Posterior surface
 2 Dorsal surface
 3 Posterior articular surface for talus
 4 Sulcus calcanei
 5 Sustentaculun tali
 6 Middle articular surface for talus
 7 Anterior articular surface for talus
 8 Articular surface for cuboid
 9 Peroneal trochlea
10 Lateral process ⎤
11 Medial process ⎦ of tuberosity
12 Plantar surface
13 Anterior tubercle
14 Groove for flexor hallucis longus tendon
15 Medial surface
16 Lateral surface
17 Tubercle for calcaneofibular ligament
18 Surface for bursa
19 Surface for tendo calcaneus
20 Surface for fibrofatty tissue
21 Medial ⎤
22 Lateral ⎦ talocalcanean ligament
23 Tibiocalcanean part of medial (deltoid) ligament
24 Interosseous talocalcanean ligament
25 Inferior extensor retinaculum
26 Cervical ligament
27 Extensor digitorum brevis
28 Calcaneocuboid part ⎤
29 Calcaneonavicular part ⎦ of bifurcate ligament

● When the talus and calcaneus are articulated the sulcus tali and sulcus calcanei form the tarsal sinus (sinus tarsi).

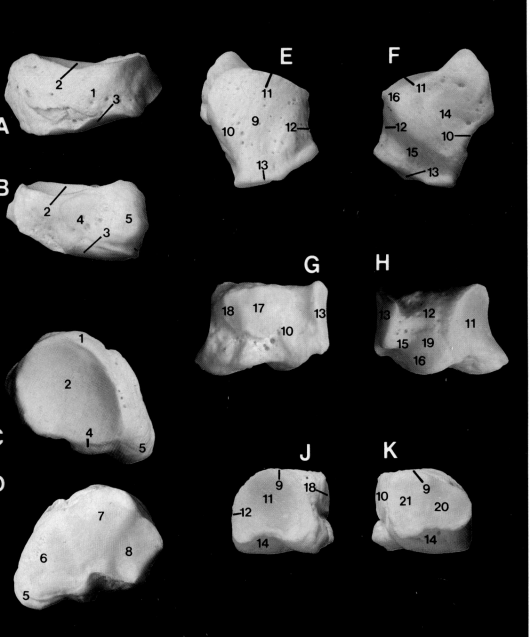

Individual foot bones

The left navicular bone

A From above	**C** Proximal aspect
B From below	**D** Distal aspect

1 Dorsal surface
2 Proximal surface for talus
3 Distal surface for cuneiforms
4 Plantar surface
5 Tuberosity
6 Facet for medial cuneiform ⎫ on
7 Facet for intermediate cuneiform ⎬ distal
8 Facet for lateral cuneiform ⎭ surface

The left cuboid bone

E From above	**H** From the lateral side
F From below	**J** Proximal aspect
G From the medial side	**K** Distal aspect

9 Dorsal surface
10 Medial surface
11 Proximal surface for calcaneus
12 Lateral surface
13 Distal surface
14 Plantar surface
15 Groove for peroneus longus tendon
16 Tuberosity
17 Surface for lateral cuneiform
18 Surface for navicular
19 Facet for sesamoid bone in peroneus longus tendon
20 Facet for fifth metatarsal ⎫ on distal
21 Facet for fourth metatarsal ⎬ surface

The articulated left cuneiform bones (medial, intermediate and lateral)

A From above **C** Proximal (navicular) aspect
B From below (for distal aspect see page 49)

The left medial cuneiform bone

D From the medial side
E From the lateral side

1 Medial surface
2 Distal surface for first metatarsal
3 Area for tendon of tibialis anterior
4 Proximal surface for navicular
5 Lateral surface
6 Surface for second metatarsal
7 Surface for intermediate cuneiform
8 Area for peroneus longus tendon

The left intermediate cuneiform bone

F From the medial side
G From the lateral side

9 Medial surface
10 Surface for medial cuneiform
11 Distal surface for second metatarsal
12 Lateral surface
13 Surface for lateral cuneiform
14 Proximal surface for navicular

The left lateral cuneiform bone

H From the medial side
J From the lateral side

15 Medial surface
16 Surfaces for second metatarsal
17 Surface for intermediate cuneiform
18 Proximal surface for navicular
19 Lateral surface
20 Surface for cuboid
21 Surface for fourth metatarsal
22 Distal surface for third metatarsal

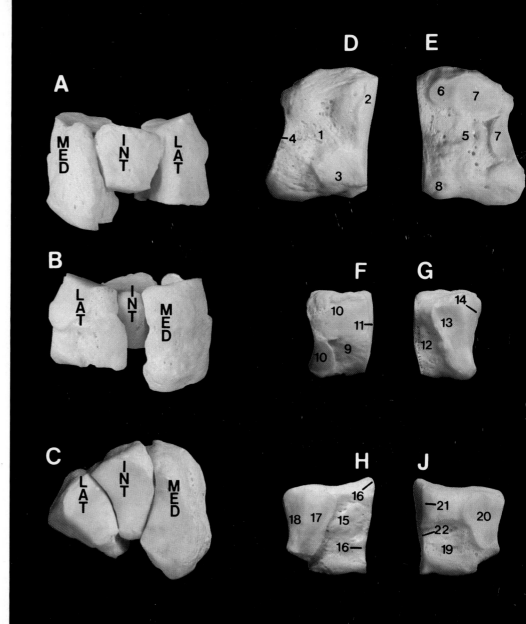

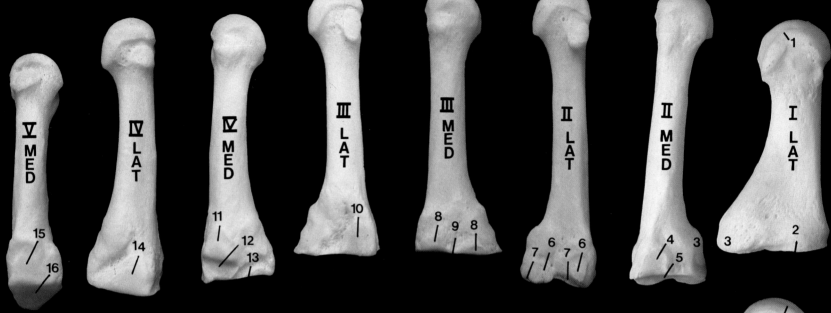

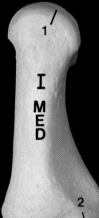

Individual foot bones

The left metatarsal bones (numbered I to V with their medial and lateral surfaces named)

1 Groove on head for sesamoid bone
2 Surface for medial cuneiform
3 Area for bursa
4 Surface for medial cuneiform
5 Surface for intermediate cuneiform
6 Surfaces for third metatarsal
7 Surfaces for lateral cuneiform
8 Surfaces for second metatarsal
9 Surface for lateral cuneiform
10 Surface for fourth metatarsal
11 Surface for third metatarsal
12 Surface for lateral cuneiform
13 Surface for cuboid
14 Surface for fifth metatarsal
15 Surface for fourth metatarsal
16 Surface for cuboid
17 Tuberosity

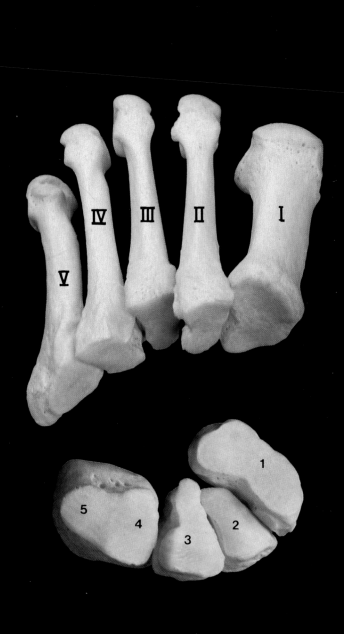

- The second, third and fourth metatarsals are longer than the first and fifth; the first is the shortest and the thickest.
- Refer to an articulated foot (page 26) and note the following:

The base of the first metatarsal articulates with the medial cuneiform. There is normally a bursa but not a joint between the bases of the first and second metatarsals.

The base of the second metatarsal articulates with all three cuneiforms and with the base of the third metatarsal. This second metatarsal base extends more proximally than the first and third bases – an interlocking device that prevents side-to-side movement.

The base of the third metatarsal articulates with the lateral cuneiform and the bases of the second and fourth metatarsals.

The base of the fourth metatarsal articulates with the lateral cuneiform and the cuboid and the base of the fifth metatarsal.

The base of the fifth metatarsal articulates with the cuboid and the base of the fourth metatarsal.

The left metatarsal bones, articulated, from above and behind (with the cuboid and cuneiform bones adjacent and turned down to show their articulating surfaces for the metatarsals)

1 Surface of medial cuneiform for first metatarsal
2 Surface of intermediate cuneiform for second metatarsal
3 Surface of lateral cuneiform for third metatarsal
4 Surface of cuboid for fourth metatarsal
5 Surface of cuboid for fifth metatarsal

- The skin of the first toe cleft is supplied by the *deep* peroneal nerve; the skin of the other clefts is supplied by the *superficial* peroneal nerve.

- The skin behind the ankle and at the back of the heel is supplied on the medial side by the saphenous nerve (from the femoral nerve) and the medial calcanean branches of the tibial nerve, and on the lateral side by the sural nerve (also from the tibial nerve).

- The saphenous nerve on the medial side of the foot supplies skin as far forward as the metatarsophalangeal joint of the great toe.

- The sural nerve on the lateral side of the foot supplies skin as far forward as the side of the fifth toe.

- The skin of the medial side of the dorsum of the foot, including the region of the medial malleolus, is part of the fourth lumbar dermatome (a dermatome is the area of skin supplied by any one spinal nerve). The fifth lumbar dermatome includes the rest of the dorsum, and the first sacral dermatome includes the lateral side of the foot and the lateral malleolar region.

- The *great* saphenous vein passes upwards *in front of the medial malleolus.*

- The *small* saphenous vein passes upwards *behind the lateral malleolus.*

Dissection of the dorsum and sides of the foot

Superficial vessels and nerves of the left foot, from the front

1 Deep fascia
2 Tendon of tibialis anterior (under fascia)
3 Tendon of extensor digitorum longus (under fascia)
4 Medial surface of tibia (under fascia)
5 Great saphenous vein
6 Saphenous nerve
7 Medial malleolus
8 Medial branch of superficial peroneal nerve
9 Lateral branch of superficial peroneal nerve
10 Lateral malleolus
11 A perforating vein
12 Proper dorsal digital nerve of great toe
13 Medial terminal branch of deep peroneal nerve
14 Dorsal venous arch
15 Dorsal digital nerve to second cleft
16 Dorsal digital nerve to third cleft
17 Dorsal digital nerve to fourth cleft
18 Sural nerve

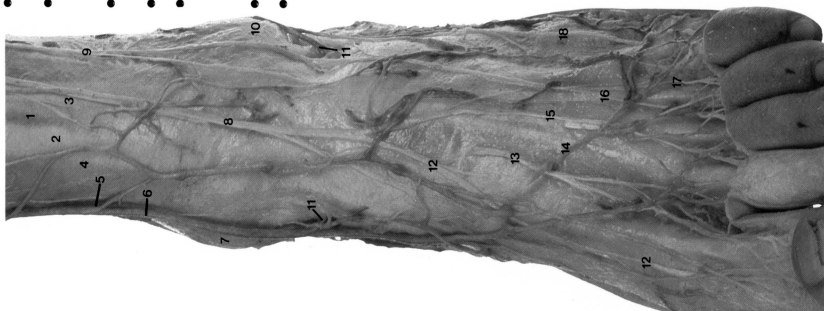

Dissection of the dorsum and sides of the foot

Superficial vessels and nerves of the left foot, from behind

1 Deep fascia
2 Sural nerve
3 Small saphenous vein
4 Posterior arch vein
5 A perforating vein
6 Tendo calcaneus (under fascia)
7 Medial malleolus
8 Medial calcanean nerve
9 Posterior surface of calcaneus
10 Fibrofatty tissue of heel
11 Lateral malleolus

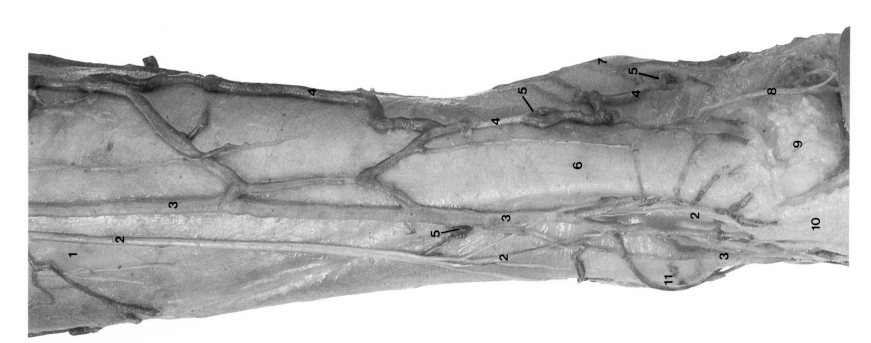

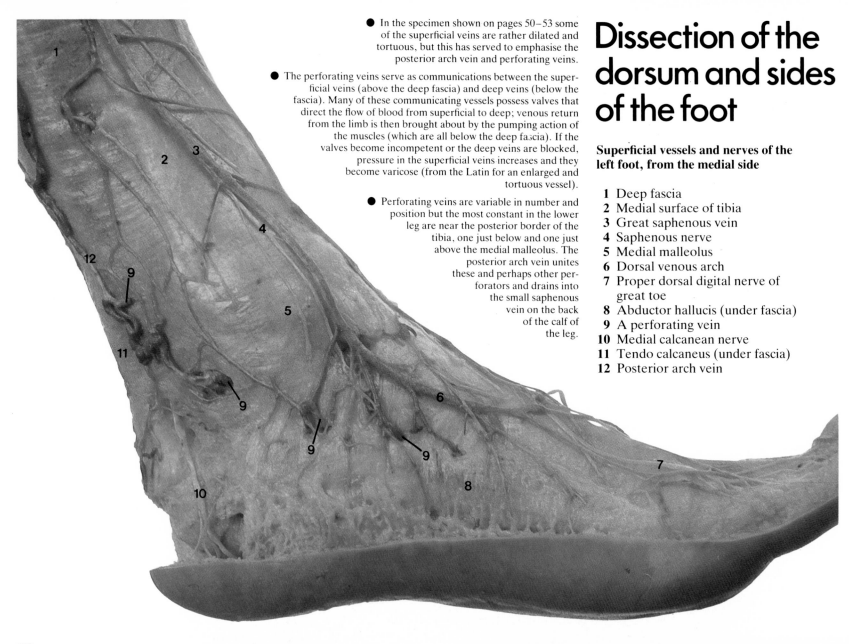

- In the specimen shown on pages 50–53 some of the superficial veins are rather dilated and tortuous, but this has served to emphasise the posterior arch vein and perforating veins.

- The perforating veins serve as communications between the superficial veins (above the deep fascia) and deep veins (below the fascia). Many of these communicating vessels possess valves that direct the flow of blood from superficial to deep; venous return from the limb is then brought about by the pumping action of the muscles (which are all below the deep fascia). If the valves become incompetent or the deep veins are blocked, pressure in the superficial veins increases and they become varicose (from the Latin for an enlarged and tortuous vessel).

- Perforating veins are variable in number and position but the most constant in the lower leg are near the posterior border of the tibia, one just below and one just above the medial malleolus. The posterior arch vein unites these and perhaps other perforators and drains into the small saphenous vein on the back of the calf of the leg.

Dissection of the dorsum and sides of the foot

Superficial vessels and nerves of the left foot, from the medial side

1 Deep fascia
2 Medial surface of tibia
3 Great saphenous vein
4 Saphenous nerve
5 Medial malleolus
6 Dorsal venous arch
7 Proper dorsal digital nerve of great toe
8 Abductor hallucis (under fascia)
9 A perforating vein
10 Medial calcanean nerve
11 Tendo calcaneus (under fascia)
12 Posterior arch vein

- The superficial veins of the dorsum include dorsal digital and dorsal metatarsal veins which join a dorsal venous arch. The ends of the arch join medial and lateral marginal veins that run upwards to become the great and small saphenous veins respectively. (In the specimen on page 52 there is no obvious medial marginal vein, but there is a lateral marginal vein on page 53.)

- The deep veins run with the deep arteries. The larger arteries in the leg are usually accompanied by a pair of veins (venae commitantes).

- Lymph vessels accompany many arteries and veins, both superficial and deep, but unless enlarged by disease they can rarely be displayed on dissection. There are no lymph nodes in the foot; most of the lymphatic drainage of the lower limb is to inguinal nodes, but some lymphatic vessels drain into six or seven nodes that lie in the fat of the popliteal fossa. (Occasionally there is a single node beside the upper end of the anterior tibial artery in front of the interosseous membrane.)

Dissection of the dorsum and sides of the foot

Superficial vessels and nerves of the left foot, from the lateral side

1 Medial branch of superficial peroneal nerve
2 Lateral branch of superficial peroneal nerve
3 Deep fascia over peroneus longus tendon
4 Sural nerve
5 Small saphenous vein
6 Tendo calcaneus (under fascia)
7 Lateral malleolus
8 A perforating vein
9 Extensor digitorum brevis (under fascia)
10 Lateral marginal vein
11 Abductor digiti minimi (under fascia)
12 Dorsal venous arch

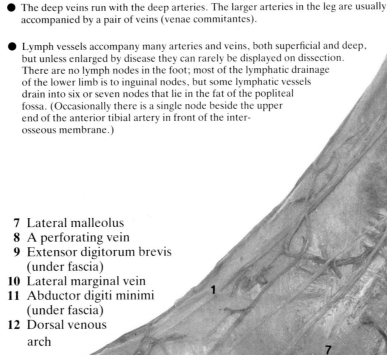

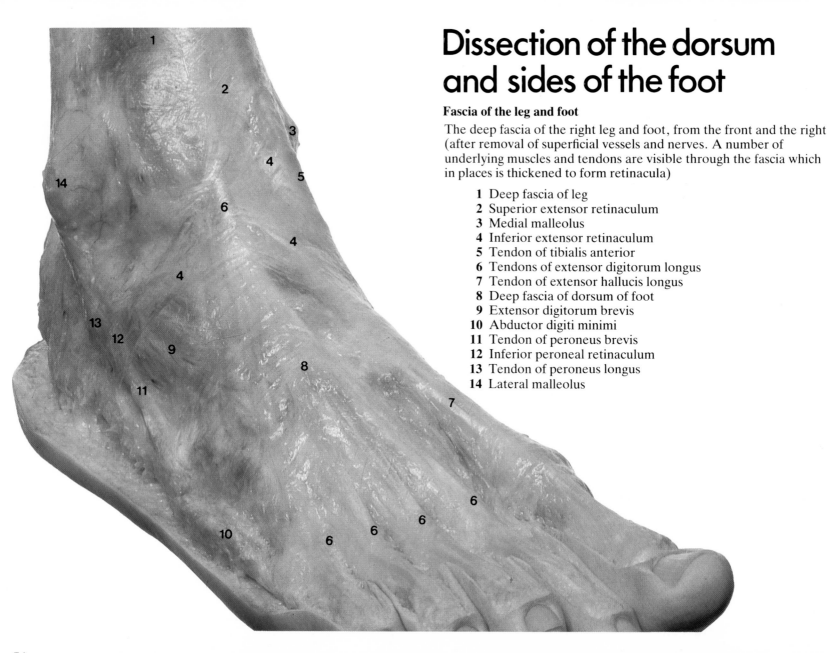

Dissection of the dorsum and sides of the foot

Fascia of the leg and foot

The deep fascia of the right leg and foot, from the front and the right (after removal of superficial vessels and nerves. A number of underlying muscles and tendons are visible through the fascia which in places is thickened to form retinacula)

1 Deep fascia of leg
2 Superior extensor retinaculum
3 Medial malleolus
4 Inferior extensor retinaculum
5 Tendon of tibialis anterior
6 Tendons of extensor digitorum longus
7 Tendon of extensor hallucis longus
8 Deep fascia of dorsum of foot
9 Extensor digitorum brevis
10 Abductor digiti minimi
11 Tendon of peroneus brevis
12 Inferior peroneal retinaculum
13 Tendon of peroneus longus
14 Lateral malleolus

- The retinacula of the ankle and foot are localised thickenings of deep fascia which keep tendons in place.

- There are two extensor retinacula (superior and inferior), a flexor retinaculum, and two peroneal retinacula (superior and inferior).

- The superior extensor retinaculum is a band about 4 cm broad, and is attached to the lower ends of the anterior borders of the tibia and fibula.

  The order of the structures that pass beneath the retinaculum and in front of the ankle joint from the medial to the lateral side is:
  Tibialis anterior tendon (with a synovial sheath)
  Extensor hallucis longus tendon (with no synovial sheath)
  Anterior tibial artery and venae commitantes
  Deep peroneal nerve
  Extensor digitorum longus tendon (with no synovial sheath)
  Peroneus tertius tendon (with no synovial sheath).

- The inferior extensor retinaculum is shaped like a letter Y lying on its side.

  The common stem of the Y is on the lateral side and is attached to the upper surface of the calcaneus in front of the sulcus calcanei. The tendons of extensor digitorum longus and peroneus tertius (with a common synovial sheath) pass beneath it.

  The upper band of the Y continues upwards and medially from the common stem over the deep peroneal nerve and anterior tibial vessels, then forms a loop to enclose the extensor hallucis longus tendon (within a synovial sheath), finally becoming attached to the medial malleolus after passing either superficial or deep to the tendon of tibialis anterior (within a synovial sheath).

  The lower band of the Y continues downwards and medially from the common stem, passing over the terminal branches of the deep peroneal nerve, the dorsalis pedis vessels and the tendons of extensor hallucis longus (within a synovial sheath) and tibialis anterior, to blend with the plantar aponeurosis overlying abductor hallucis.

Dissection of the dorsum and sides of the foot

Muscles, nerves and vessels of the right foot, from the front

(The synovial sheaths of tendons have been emphasised by blue tissue)

1 Medial surface of tibia
2 Tibialis anterior
3 Extensor hallucis longus
4 Extensor digitorum longus
5 Subcutaneous surface of fibula
6 Peroneus brevis
7 Superior extensor retinaculum
8 Lateral malleolus
9 Inferior extensor retinaculum
10 Medial malleolus
11 Tibialis posterior
12 Extensor hallucis brevis
13 Extensor digitorum brevis
14 Dorsalis pedis artery
15 First dorsal interosseous
16 Second dorsal interosseous
17 Third dorsal interosseous
18 Fourth dorsal interosseous
19 Peroneus tertius
20 Dorsal digital expansion

● Extensor digitorum longus has four tendons which pass to the second, third, fourth and fifth toes.

● Extensor digitorum brevis has four tendons which pass to the great, second, third and fourth toes. The part of the muscle that serves the great toe is known as extensor hallucis brevis.

● The dorsal digital expansions (extensor expansions) are derived from the tendons of extensor digitorum longus as they pass on to the dorsum of the proximal phalanges, over the metatarsophalangeal joints. They are each triangular in shape with the apex directed distally.

On the second, third and fourth toes the basal angles receive tendons from two interossei and one lumbrical muscle, and the central part of the base receives a tendon of extensor digitorum brevis. On the fifth toe one interosseous and one lumbrical tendon are attached.

The central part of the apex is inserted into the base of the middle phalanx, while two collateral parts run farther forward to be inserted into the base of the distal phalanx.

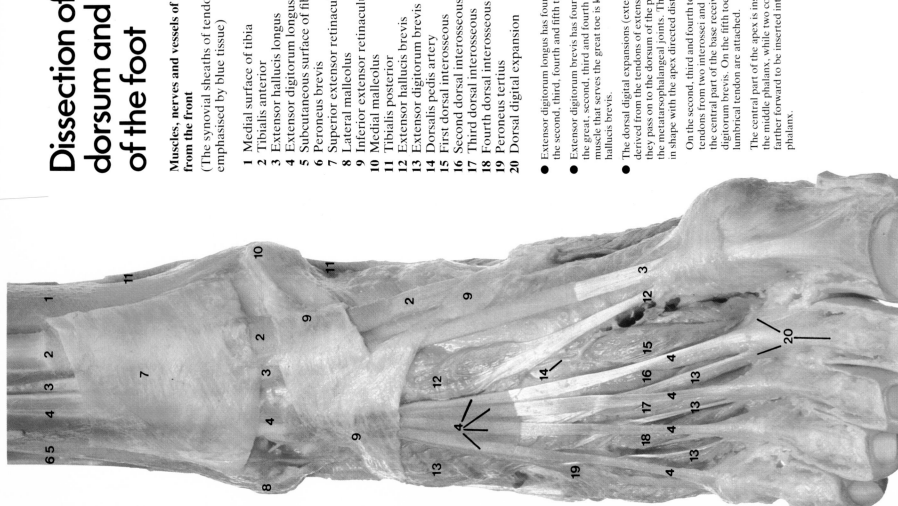

Dissection of the dorsum and sides of the foot

Muscles, nerves and vessels of the right foot, from behind

(The synovial sheaths of tendons have been emphasised by blue tissue)

1 Peroneus longus
2 Soleus
3 Sural nerve
4 Tendo calcaneus
5 Lateral malleolus
6 Superior peroneal retinaculum
7 Inferior peroneal retinaculum
8 Posterior surface of calcaneus
9 Flexor retinaculum
10 Medial malleolus
11 Tibialis posterior
12 Flexor digitorum longus
13 Posterior tibial artery and venae commitantes
14 Tibial nerve
15 Flexor hallucis longus
16 Medial calcanean nerve
17 Plantaris tendon

● In this specimen the muscle fibres of peroneus longus extend unusually low.

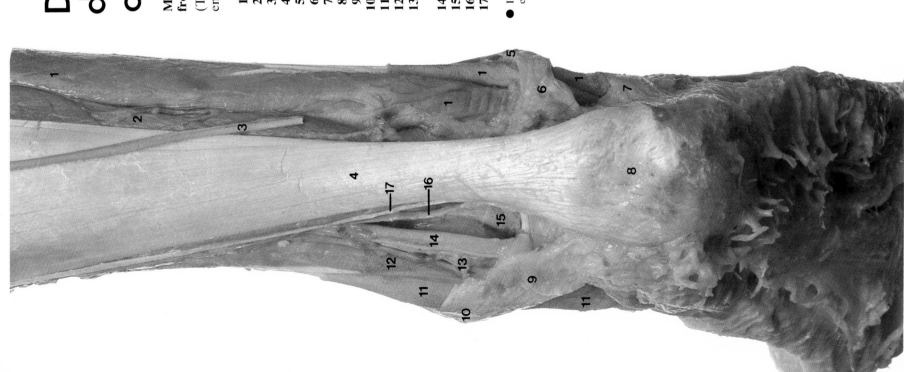

Dissection of the dorsum and sides of the foot

Muscles, nerves and vessels of the right foot, from the medial side

(The synovial sheaths of tendons have been emphasised by blue tissue)

1 Medial surface of tibia
2 Tibialis posterior
3 Flexor digitorum longus
4 Posterior tibial artery and venae commitantes
5 Tibial nerve
6 Flexor hallucis longus
7 Soleus
8 Plantaris tendon
9 Tendo calcaneus
10 Medial calcanean nerve
11 Posterior surface of calcaneus
12 Flexor retinaculum
13 Medial malleolus
14 Abductor hallucis
15 Inferior extensor retinaculum
16 Tibialis anterior
17 Extensor hallucis longus

● The flexor retinaculum passes from the medial malleolus to the medial process of the tuberosity of the calcaneus.

Deep to the retinaculum are four connective tissue compartments – three for tendons and one for neurovascular structures. The order of the structures behind the medial malleolus from before backwards is:

Tibialis posterior tendon (within a synovial sheath)
Flexor digitorum longus (within a synovial sheath)
Posterior tibial artery and venae commitantes
Tibial nerve
Flexor hallucis longus tendon (within a synovial sheath).

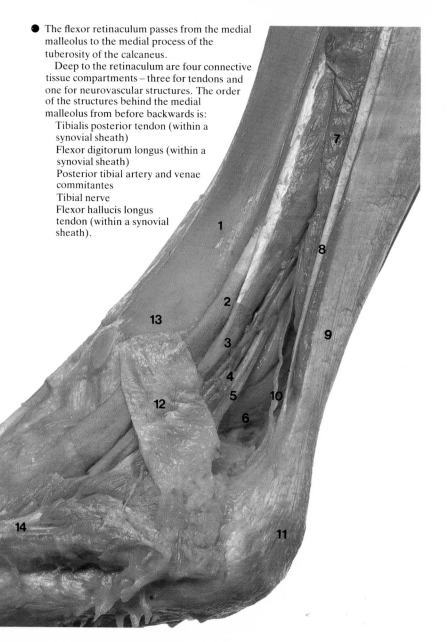

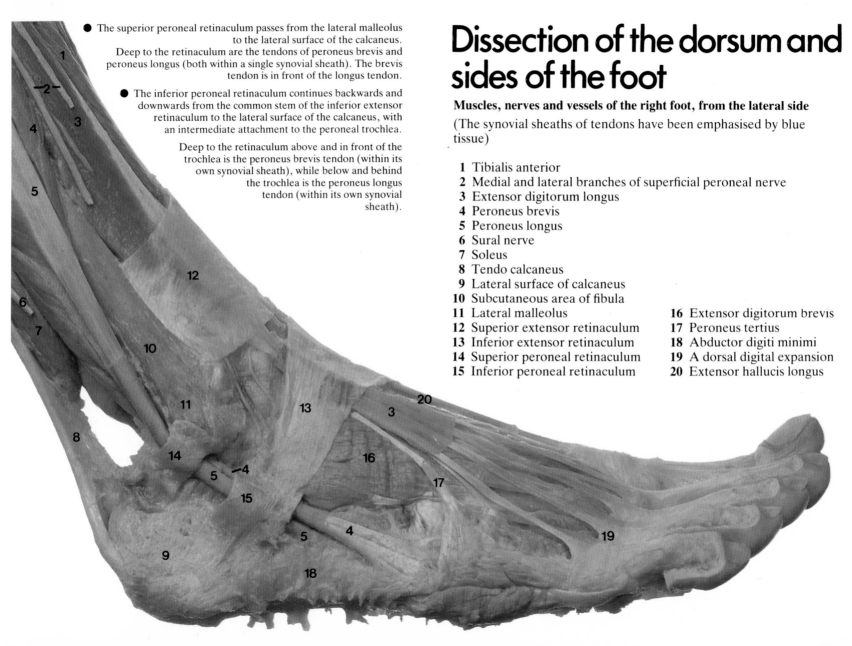

- The superior peroneal retinaculum passes from the lateral malleolus to the lateral surface of the calcaneus. Deep to the retinaculum are the tendons of peroneus brevis and peroneus longus (both within a single synovial sheath). The brevis tendon is in front of the longus tendon.

- The inferior peroneal retinaculum continues backwards and downwards from the common stem of the inferior extensor retinaculum to the lateral surface of the calcaneus, with an intermediate attachment to the peroneal trochlea.

  Deep to the retinaculum above and in front of the trochlea is the peroneus brevis tendon (within its own synovial sheath), while below and behind the trochlea is the peroneus longus tendon (within its own synovial sheath).

Dissection of the dorsum and sides of the foot

Muscles, nerves and vessels of the right foot, from the lateral side

(The synovial sheaths of tendons have been emphasised by blue tissue)

1 Tibialis anterior
2 Medial and lateral branches of superficial peroneal nerve
3 Extensor digitorum longus
4 Peroneus brevis
5 Peroneus longus
6 Sural nerve
7 Soleus
8 Tendo calcaneus
9 Lateral surface of calcaneus
10 Subcutaneous area of fibula
11 Lateral malleolus
12 Superior extensor retinaculum
13 Inferior extensor retinaculum
14 Superior peroneal retinaculum
15 Inferior peroneal retinaculum
16 Extensor digitorum brevis
17 Peroneus tertius
18 Abductor digiti minimi
19 A dorsal digital expansion
20 Extensor hallucis longus

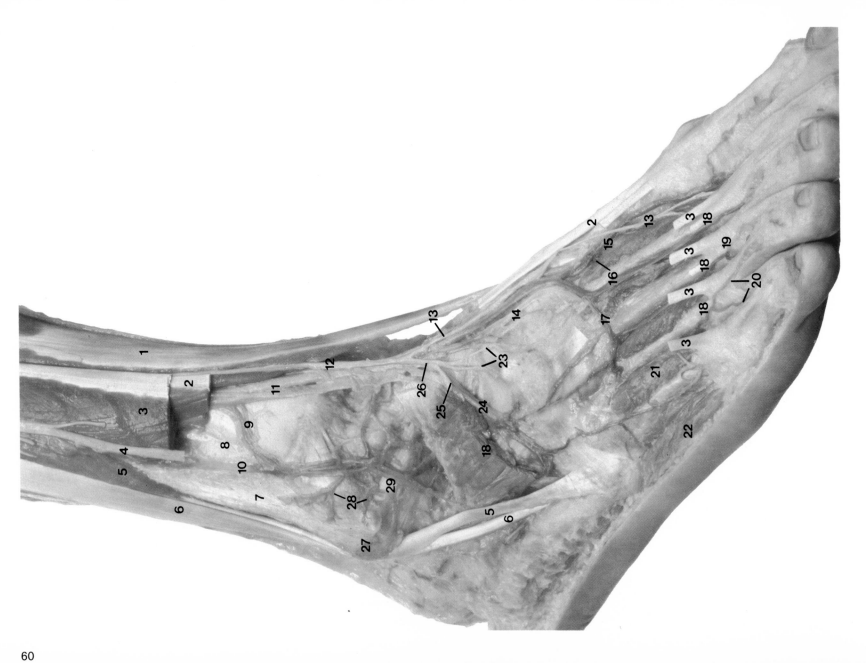

60

Dissection of the dorsum and sides of the foot

Deep nerves and vessels of the dorsum of the right foot, from the front and the right

(A number of veins accompanying arteries have been preserved.)

1 Tibialis anterior
2 Extensor hallucis longus
3 Extensor digitorum longus
4 Lateral branch of superficial peroneal nerve
5 Peroneus brevis
6 Peroneus longus
7 Subcutaneous surface of fibula
8 Interosseous membrane
9 Lateral malleolar vessels
10 Perforating branch of peroneal artery
11 Anterior tibial vessels
12 Deep peroneal nerve
13 Medial terminal branch of 12
14 Dorsalis pedis artery
15 First dorsal metatarsal artery
16 Deep plantar artery
17 Arcuate artery
18 Extensor digitorum brevis
19 Dorsal digital expansion
20 Dorsal digital artery
21 Fourth dorsal interosseous
22 Abductor digiti minimi
23 Interosseous branch of 26
24 Lateral tarsal vessels
25 Nerve to extensor digitorum brevis
26 Lateral terminal branch of 12
27 Lateral malleolus
28 Lateral malleolar arterial rete
29 Anterior talofibular ligament

● As the anterior tibial artery crosses the lower margin of the tibia at the ankle joint it becomes the dorsalis pedis artery.

● After giving off medial and lateral tarsal branches the dorsalis pedis artery ends by dividing into the first dorsal metatarsal and the arcuate arteries.

● The first dorsal metatarsal artery gives off a deep plantar (perforating) branch that passes into the sole between the two heads of the first dorsal interosseous muscle to complete the plantar arch with the deep part of the lateral plantar artery.

● The arcuate artery gives off the other three dorsal metatarsal arteries, and all the metatarsal arteries give dorsal digital branches.

● Sometimes the perforating branch of the peroneal artery, which anastomoses with the lateral tarsal and arcuate arteries, is large and replaces the dorsalis pedis.

● Theoretically each side of each toe has a dorsal digital artery and a plantar digital artery (page 67) but the individual vessels soon become merged into an anastomotic network.

● For a summary of the branches of the dorsalis pedis artery see page 92.

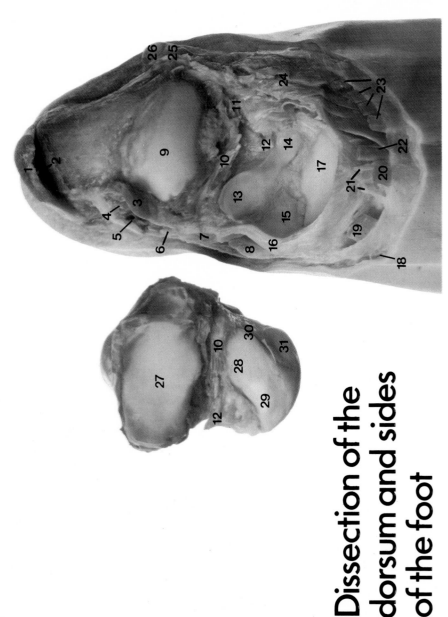

Dissection of the dorsum and sides of the foot

The left foot, from above, with the talus removed and turned upside down (so disarticulating the talocalcanean and talocalcaneonavicular joints)

1 Tendo calcaneus
2 Bursa
3 Flexor hallucis longus
4 Lateral plantar nerve
5 Posterior tibial vessels
6 Medial plantar nerve
7 Flexor digitorum longus
8 Tibialis posterior
9 Posterior articular surface of calcaneus
10 Interosseous talocalcanean ligament
11 Inferior extensor retinaculum
12 Cervical ligament
13 Middle ⎫ articular surface of calcaneus
14 Anterior ⎭
15 Cartilage in plantar calcaneonavicular (spring) ligament
16 Medial (deltoid) ligament of ankle joint
17 Posterior articular surface of navicular
18 Great saphenous vein
19 Tibialis anterior
20 Extensor hallucis longus
21 Deep peroneal nerve
22 Dorsalis pedis artery
23 Extensor digitorum longus
24 Extensor digitorum brevis
25 Peroneus brevis
26 Peroneus longus
27 Posterior ⎫ calcanean articular surface of talus
28 Middle ⎬
29 Anterior ⎭
30 Surface for plantar calcaneonavicular (spring) ligament
31 Surface for navicular

● Apart from the joints of the toes, the most important joints of the rest of the foot are those related to the talus.

● Above the talus is the ankle joint (properly known as the talocrural joint), between the trochlear surface of the talus and the lower ends of the tibia and fibula.

● Below the talus there are two separate joints. Towards the back is the talocalcanean joint (alternatively known as the subtalar joint – but see below), between the posterior articular surfaces of the lower part of the talus and upper part of the calcaneus. In front is the talocalcaneonavicular joint, which is a two-part joint between the front of the head of the talus and the navicular (the talonavicular part of this joint), and the articulations of the under surface of the talus with the anterior and middle facets on the upper surface of the calcaneus and the upper surface of the plantar calcaneonavicular (spring) ligament (the talocalcanean part of this joint).

● Unfortunately there is some confusion of terminology, for clinicians frequently use 'subtalar joint' as a collective name for *both* joints beneath the talus, not just the posterior one.

Dissection of the sole of the foot

The left plantar aponeurosis and cutaneous nerves

1 Plantar digital nerve
2 Superficial transverse metatarsal ligament
3 Superficial layer of digital band of aponeurosis
4 Deep layer of digital band of aponeurosis
5 Transverse fibres of aponeurosis
6 Proper plantar digital nerve of great toe
7 Common plantar digital branch of medial plantar nerve
8 Common plantar digital branch of lateral plantar nerve
9 Central part of aponeurosis overlying flexor digitorum brevis
10 Medial part of aponeurosis overlying abductor hallucis
11 Lateral part of aponeurosis overlying abductor digiti minimi
12 Medial calcanean nerve
13 Medial process of tuberosity of calcaneus
14 Proper plantar digital nerve of fifth toe

● **Nerve supplies in the sole**
 Cutaneous: the medial plantar nerve supplies the medial part of the sole and the medial three and a half toes; the lateral plantar nerve supplies the lateral part of the sole and the lateral one and a half toes.
 Muscular: the medial plantar nerve supplies abductor hallucis, flexor hallucis brevis, flexor digitorum brevis and the first lumbrical; the lateral plantar nerve supplies all the other small muscles of the sole.

 For details of nerve branches see page 92.

● The skin under the heel and on the lateral part of the sole is part of the first sacral dermatome, with the fifth lumbar dermatome including the central part of the sole and the fourth lumbar dermatome including the medial part.

● The superficial surface of the plantar aponeurosis is not smooth but has numerous fibrous septa forming loculations that hold the fatty subcutaneous tissues in place when weight-bearing. They are well shown towards the back and sides of the dissection illustrated here.

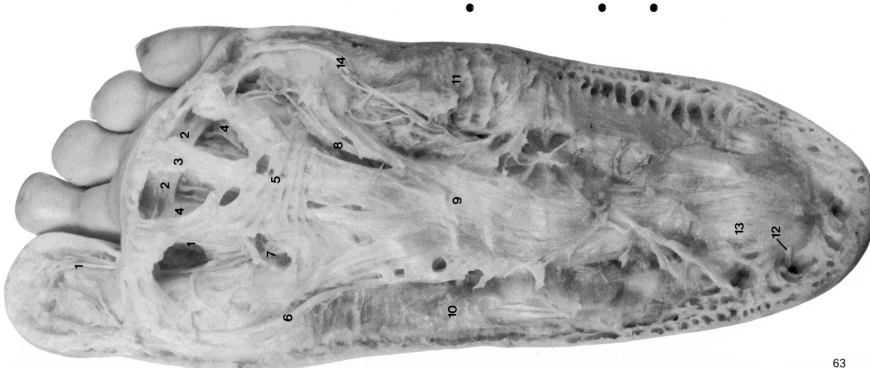

Dissection of the sole of the foot

The left sole: the first layer of muscles (after removal of the plantar aponeurosis)

1 Proper plantar digital nerve of great toe
2 Proper plantar digital nerves of first cleft
3 Superficial transverse metatarsal ligament
4 Fibrous flexor sheath
5 First lumbrical
6 Second lumbrical
7 Third lumbrical
8 Fourth lumbrical
9 Third plantar metatarsal artery
10 A superficial digital branch of medial plantar artery
11 Fourth common plantar digital nerve
12 Fourth dorsal interosseous
13 Third plantar interosseous
14 Proper plantar digital nerve of fifth toe
15 Flexor digiti minimi brevis
16 Abductor digiti minimi
17 Deep branch of lateral plantar nerve
18 Lateral plantar artery
19 Flexor digitorum brevis
20 Plantar aponeurosis
21 Abductor hallucis
22 Flexor hallucis brevis
23 Flexor hallucis longus
24 First common plantar digital nerve

● The muscles of the sole are usually classified in four layers, as seen in progressively deep dissection, but a medial, lateral and intermediate grouping may be functionally more useful:
Medial group, for the great toe: abductor hallucis, flexor hallucis brevis, adductor hallucis, with the tendon of flexor hallucis longus.
Lateral group, for the fifth toe: abductor digiti minimi, and flexor digiti minimi brevis.
Intermediate group, for the second to fifth toes: flexor digitorum brevis, flexor accessorius, the tendons of flexor digitorum longus and the lumbricals, and the interossei.

● The medial and lateral plantar nerves and vessels pass between the first and second layers; the deep parts of the lateral plantar nerve and vessels pass between the third and fourth layers, curling medially and deeply round the lateral border of flexor accessorius.

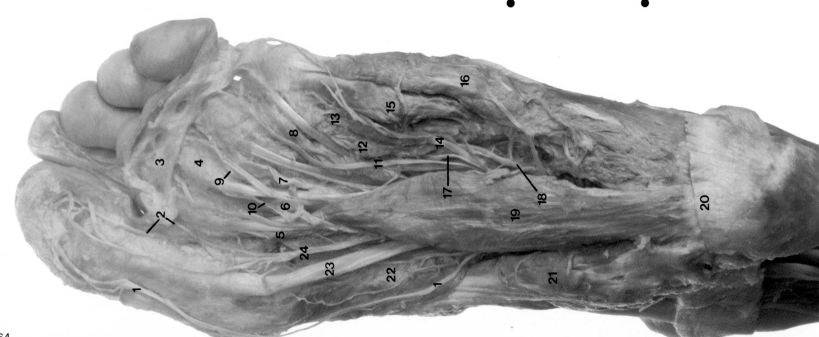

Dissection of the sole of the foot

The left sole: the second layer of muscles

(The synovial sheaths of tendons in the sole have been emphasised by blue tissue)

1 Flexor hallucis longus
2 Fibrous flexor sheath
3 Flexor digitorum brevis
4 Flexor digitorum longus
5 Proper plantar digital nerve of great toe
6 Flexor hallucis brevis
7 First lumbrical
8 Second lumbrical
9 Third lumbrical
10 Fourth lumbrical
11 Fourth plantar metatarsal artery
12 Fourth dorsal interosseous
13 Third plantar interosseous
14 Proper plantar digital nerve of fifth toe
15 Flexor digiti minimi brevis
16 Abductor digiti minimi
17 Plantar arch
18 Deep branch of lateral plantar nerve
19 Flexor accessorius
20 Lateral plantar artery
21 Nerve to abductor digiti minimi
22 Lateral plantar nerve
23 Fourth common plantar digital nerve
24 Nerve to flexor accessorius
25 Nerve to flexor digitorum brevis
26 Medial plantar artery overlying nerve
27 Abductor hallucis
28 Nerve to flexor hallucis brevis
29 First common plantar digital nerve
30 Nerve to first lumbrical

● Although flexor hallucis longus passes to the great toe on the *medial* side of the foot it arises from the fibula on the *lateral* side of the leg. The tendon crosses over in the sole, deep to flexor digitorum longus.

● First layer: abductor hallucis, flexor digitorum brevis and abductor digiti minimi.

● Second layer: flexor accessorius and the four lumbricals (with the tendons of flexor digitorum lingus and flexor hallucis longus).

● Third layer: flexor hallucis brevis, adductor hallucis and flexor digiti minimi brevis.

● Fourth layer: plantar and dorsal interossei (with the tendons of tibialis posterior and peroneus longus).

● The successive layers do not completely obscure one another; for example, the third plantar and fourth dorsal interossei of the fourth layer are seen as soon as the plantar aponeurosis is removed. (The layers refer to layers of *muscles*; the plantar *aponeurosis* is not itself the first layer – it overlies the first layer.)

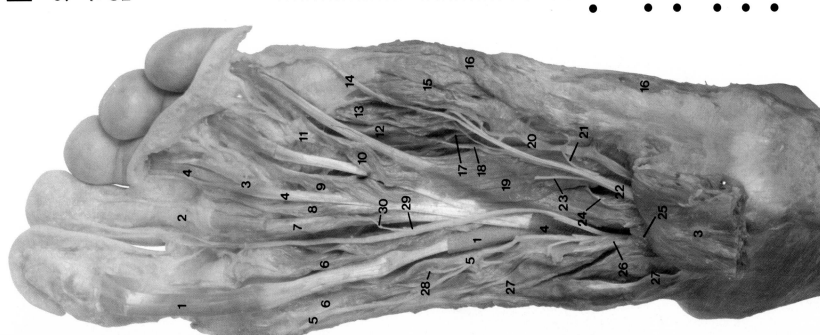

Dissection of the sole of the foot

The left sole: the third layer of muscles

1 Flexor hallucis longus
2 Flexor digitorum longus
3 Flexor digitorum brevis
4 Fibrous flexor sheath
5 Long vinculum
6 Transverse head ⎤
7 Oblique head   ⎦ of adductor hallucis
8 Flexor hallucis brevis
9 Second plantar interosseous
10 Fourth dorsal interosseous
11 Third plantar interosseous
12 Fourth plantar metatarsal artery
13 Abductor digiti minimi
14 Flexor digiti minimi brevis
15 Nerve to flexor digiti minimi brevis
16 Plantar arch
17 Deep branch of lateral plantar nerve
18 Nerve to adductor hallucis
19 Lateral plantar artery
20 Lateral plantar nerve
21 Flexor accessorius
22 Medial plantar nerve
23 Abductor hallucis
24 Medial plantar artery
25 Nerve to abductor hallucis
26 Tuberosity of navicular
27 Tibialis anterior

- For a summary of the medial and lateral plantar nerves see page 92.

- The third common plantar digital nerve (from the medial plantar nerve) frequently has a communicating branch with the (fourth) common plantar digital branch of the lateral plantar nerve, but it was not present in the specimens dissected here.

- Both here and on pages 65 and 67 branches of the lateral plantar nerve to various interosseous muscles can be seen but have been left unlabelled.

- The plantar arch is the deep continuation of the lateral plantar artery, which is the larger terminal branch of the posterior tibial artery. The arch is completed by anastomosis with the deep plantar (perforating) branch of the first dorsal metatarsal artery.

  The arch gives off four plantar metatarsal arteries which divide to give plantar digital branches to the sides of adjacent toes. There are separate branches for the medial side of the great toe and lateral side of the fifth toe.

- The medial plantar artery, smaller than the lateral and subject to considerable variation, does not take part directly in the formation of the arch. It usually anastomoses with the plantar digital branch to the medial side of the great toe; and gives off superficial digital branches that anastomose with the first three plantar metatarsal arteries.

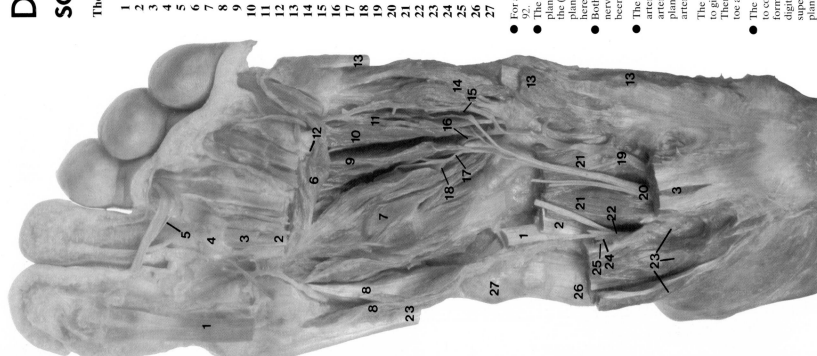

Dissection of the sole of the foot

The left sole: the fourth layer of muscles

(The synovial sheaths of the first and second toes have been emphasised by blue tissue)

1 Flexor hallucis longus
2 Fibrous flexor sheath
3 Flexor digitorum longus
4 Flexor digitorum brevis
5 First dorsal interosseous
6 Second dorsal interosseous
7 First plantar interosseous
8 Third dorsal interosseous
9 Second plantar interosseous
10 Fourth dorsal interosseous
11 Third plantar interosseous
12 Flexor digiti minimi brevis
13 Abductor digiti minimi
14 First plantar metatarsal artery
15 Second plantar metatarsal artery
16 Third plantar metatarsal artery
17 Fourth plantar metatarsal artery
18 Plantar arch
19 Deep branch of lateral plantar nerve
20 Lateral plantar artery
21 Lateral plantar nerve
22 Medial plantar nerve
23 Medial plantar artery
24 Peroneus longus
25 Tibialis anterior
26 Tuberosity of navicular
27 Tibialis posterior
28 Abductor hallucis
29 Flexor accessorius

● Viewed from the sole, both plantar *and* dorsal interossei are visible; they lie side by side, not (as might be expected from their names) with the plantar group completely overlying and obscuring the dorsal. (But on the dorsum only dorsal interossei are seen between the metatarsals – as on page 56.)

The *plantar* interossei *adduct* toes and the *dorsal* interossei *abduct* them, the reference line or axis for these movements being the line of the second toe. The mnemonics PAD and DAB are the usual aid to recalling which group does what.

The great toe and the fifth toe each have their own abductor muscle; the great toe also has its own adductor to draw it nearer the second toe. It follows that there must be a plantar interosseous for each of the third, fourth and fifth toes so that they can be adducted towards the axial line.

The second toe has no plantar interosseous but it has two dorsal interossei, one on each side so that it can be abducted to either side of its own neutral position.

The third and fourth toes both have one of each interosseous.

For other and probably more important actions of the interossei see page 79.

For a summary of the medial and lateral plantar arteries see page 93.

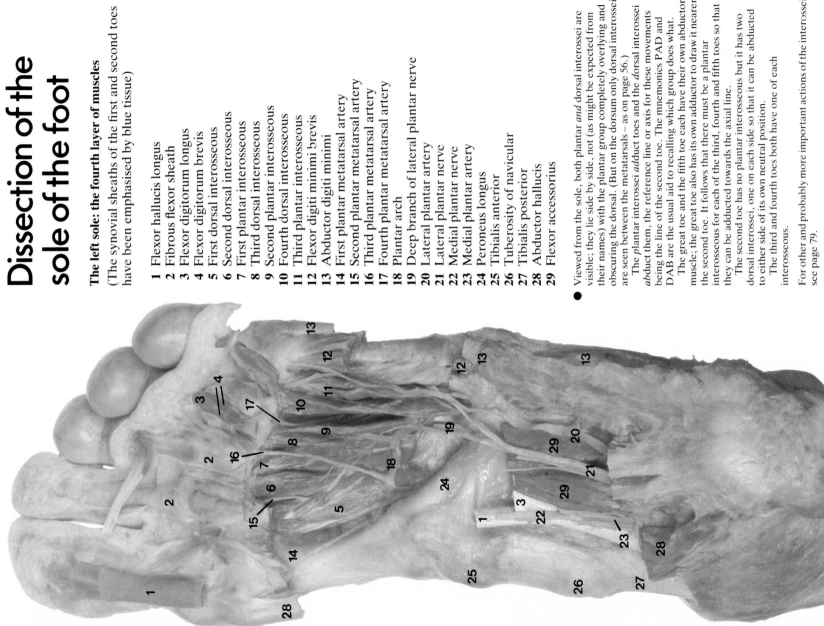

67

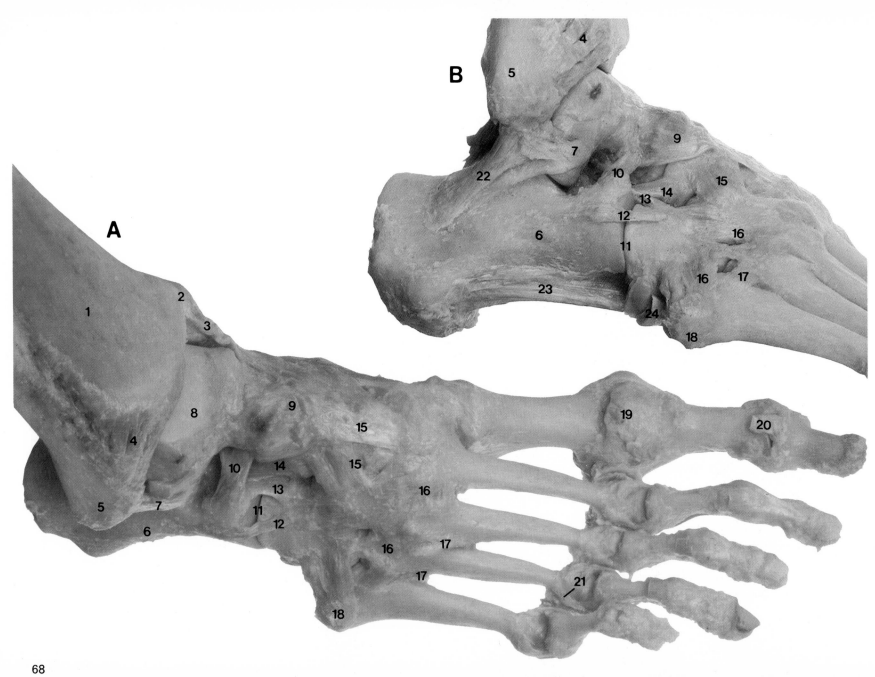

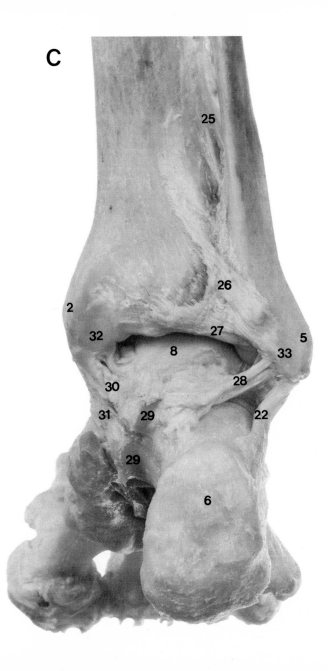

C

25

26

2

32

27

5

8

33

30

28

31

29

22

29

6

Ligaments of the foot

Ligaments of the right foot

A From the right and above
B From the lateral side
C From behind

1 Tibia
2 Medial malleolus
3 Medial (deltoid) ligament of ankle joint
4 Anterior tibiofibular ligament
5 Lateral malleolus
6 Calcaneus
7 Anterior talofibular ligament
8 Trochlear surface of talus (ankle joint capsule removed)
9 Head of talus (under capsule of talonavicular part of talocalcaneonavicular joint)
10 Cervical ligament
11 Calcaneocuboid joint
12 Dorsal calcaneocuboid ligament
13 Calcaneocuboid part ⎤
14 Calcaneonavicular part ⎦ of bifurcate ligament
15 Dorsal cuneonavicular ligaments
16 Dorsal tarsometatarsal ligaments
17 Dorsal metatarsal ligaments
18 Tuberosity of base of fifth metatarsal
19 Capsule of first metatarsophalangeal joint
20 Tendon of extensor hallucis longus
21 Collateral ligament
22 Calcaneofibular ligament
23 Long plantar ligament
24 Tendon of peroneus longus
25 Interosseous membrane
26 Posterior tibiofibular ligament
27 Tibial slip of 28
28 Posterior talofibular ligament
29 Groove for flexor hallucis longus tendon
30 Posterior tibiotalal part ⎤
31 Tibiocalcanean part ⎦ of medial (deltoid) ligament
32 Groove for tibialis posterior tendon
33 Groove for peroneus brevis tendon

Ligaments of the foot

Ligaments of the right foot, from the medial side

1 Medial malleolus
2 Posterior tibiotalal part ⎤
3 Tibiocalcanean part ⎥
4 Anterior tibiotalal part ⎬ of medial (deltoid) ligament
5 Tibionavicular part ⎦
6 Sustentaculum tali
7 Tibialis posterior
8 Tuberosity of navicular
9 Long plantar ligament
10 Dorsal cuneonavicular ligament
11 Talonavicular ligament
12 Dorsal ligaments of first tarsometatarsal joint
13 Tibialis anterior
14 Capsule ⎤
15 Collateral ligament ⎦ of first metatarsophalangeal joint
16 Sesamoid bone
17 Flexor hallucis longus
18 Collateral ligament of interphalangeal joint
19 Extensor hallucis longus

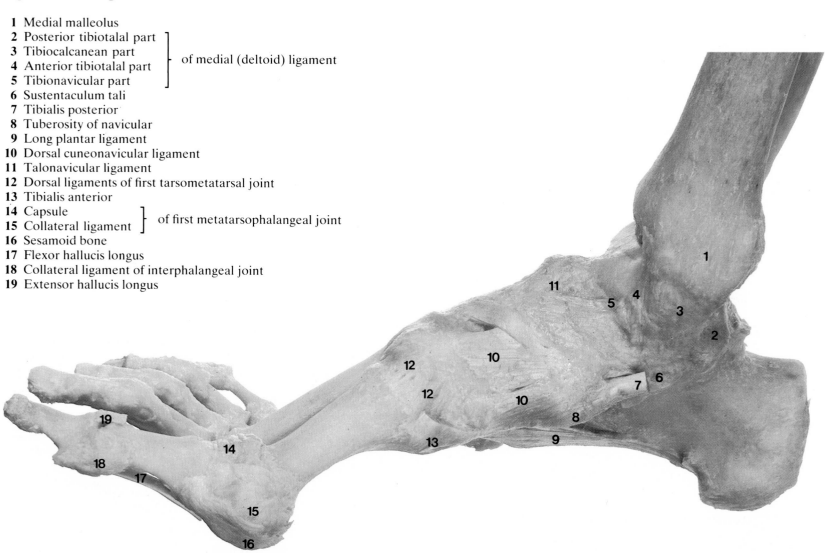

Ligaments of the foot

Ligaments of the sole of the right foot (the part of the long plantar ligament that covers the tendon of peroneus longus has been removed)

1 Flexor digitorum longus
2 Flexor digitorum brevis
3 Fibrous flexor sheath
4 Deep transverse metatarsal ligament
5 Flexor hallucis longus
6 Plantar ligament of first metatarsophalangeal joint
7 Plantar tarsometatarsal ligament
8 Peroneus longus
9 Long plantar ligament
10 Tuberosity of base of fifth metatarsal
11 Plantar cuneonavicular ligament
12 Slip from tibialis posterior
13 Plantar calcaneocuboid (short plantar) ligament
14 Plantar calcaneonavicular (spring) ligament
15 Tuberosity of navicular
16 Tibialis posterior
17 Sustentaculum tali
18 Groove for flexor hallucis longus

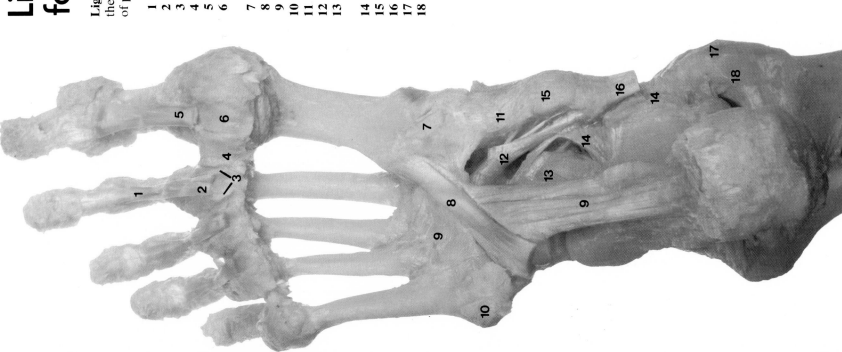

Sections of the foot

Sagittal sections of the right foot

A Through the medial part of the talus, sustentaculum tali and the great toe, from the lateral side

B Through the centre of the talus, medial part of the calcaneus and the great toe, from the lateral side (in a different foot from A)

1 Tibia
2 Tibialis posterior
3 Flexor digitorum longus
4 Tibial nerve
5 Flexor hallucis longus
6 Talus
7 Sustentaculum tali
8 Plantar calcaneonavicular (spring) ligament
9 Navicular
10 Tibialis anterior
11 Medial cuneiform
12 First metatarsal
13 Extensor hallucis longus
14 Proximal phalanx
15 Distal phalanx
16 Sesamoid bone
17 Flexor hallucis brevis

72

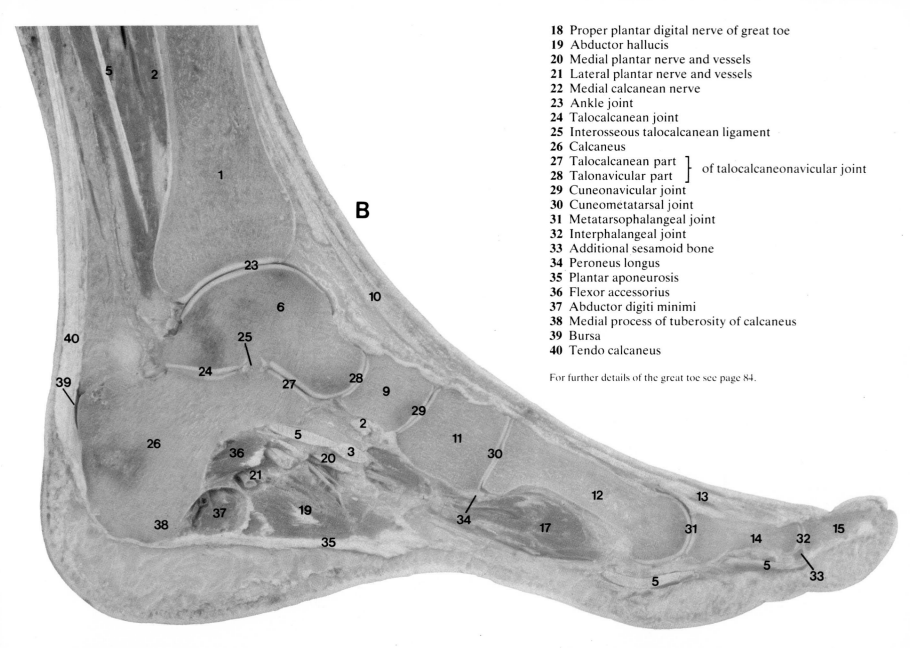

18 Proper plantar digital nerve of great toe
19 Abductor hallucis
20 Medial plantar nerve and vessels
21 Lateral plantar nerve and vessels
22 Medial calcanean nerve
23 Ankle joint
24 Talocalcanean joint
25 Interosseous talocalcanean ligament
26 Calcaneus
27 Talocalcanean part ⎱ of talocalcaneonavicular joint
28 Talonavicular part ⎰
29 Cuneonavicular joint
30 Cuneometatarsal joint
31 Metatarsophalangeal joint
32 Interphalangeal joint
33 Additional sesamoid bone
34 Peroneus longus
35 Plantar aponeurosis
36 Flexor accessorius
37 Abductor digiti minimi
38 Medial process of tuberosity of calcaneus
39 Bursa
40 Tendo calcaneus

For further details of the great toe see page 84.

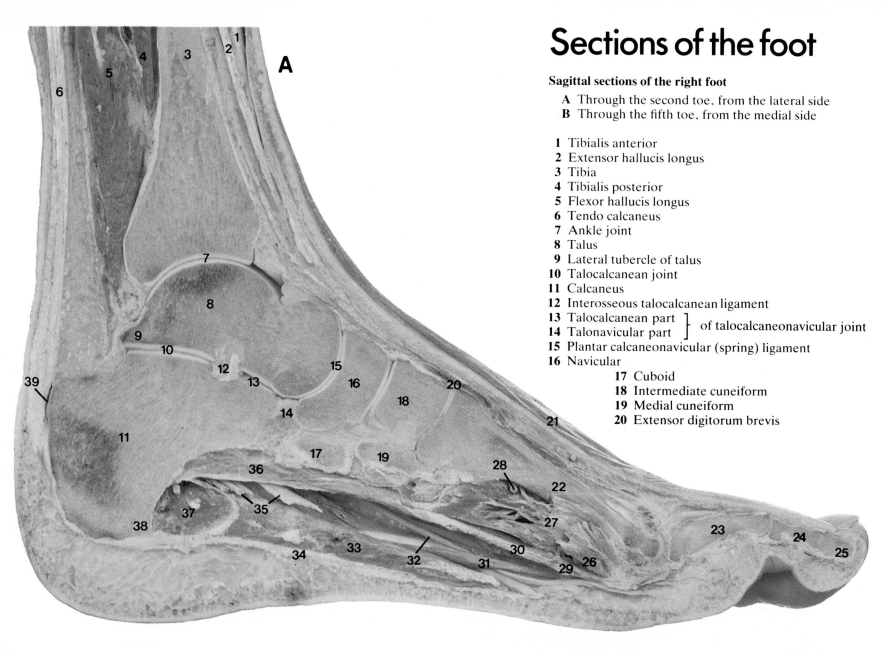

Sections of the foot

Sagittal sections of the right foot

  A Through the second toe, from the lateral side
  B Through the fifth toe, from the medial side

 1 Tibialis anterior
 2 Extensor hallucis longus
 3 Tibia
 4 Tibialis posterior
 5 Flexor hallucis longus
 6 Tendo calcaneus
 7 Ankle joint
 8 Talus
 9 Lateral tubercle of talus
 10 Talocalcanean joint
 11 Calcaneus
 12 Interosseous talocalcanean ligament
 13 Talocalcanean part ⎤
 14 Talonavicular part ⎦ of talocalcaneonavicular joint
 15 Plantar calcaneonavicular (spring) ligament
 16 Navicular
   17 Cuboid
   18 Intermediate cuneiform
   19 Medial cuneiform
   20 Extensor digitorum brevis

21 Extensor digitorum longus tendon to second toe
22 Second metatarsal
23 Proximal ⎫
24 Middle ⎬ phalanx of second toe
25 Distal ⎭
26 Transverse head ⎫ of adductor hallucis
27 Oblique head ⎭
28 Plantar arch
29 Second lumbrical overlying flexor digitorum longus tendon to second toe
30 Flexor digitorum longus tendon to third toe
31 Flexor digitorum brevis tendon to second toe
32 Second common plantar digital nerve
33 Flexor digitorum brevis
34 Plantar aponeurosis
35 Lateral plantar nerve and vessels
36 Flexor accessorius
37 Abductor digiti minimi
38 Medial process of tuberosity of calcaneus
39 Bursa
40 Lateral branch of superficial peroneal nerve
41 Fibula
42 Peroneus longus
43 Peroneus brevis
44 Lateral process of tuberosity of calcaneus
45 Calcaneocuboid joint
46 Cuboideometatarsal joint
47 Fifth metatarsal
48 Flexor digiti minimi brevis
49 Metatarsophalangeal joint of fifth toe

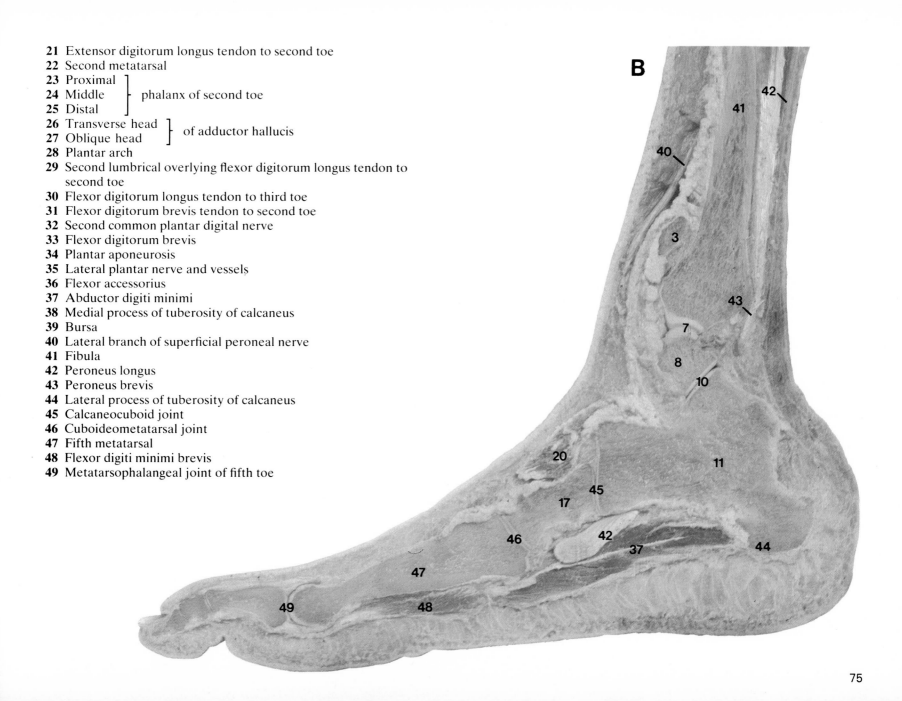

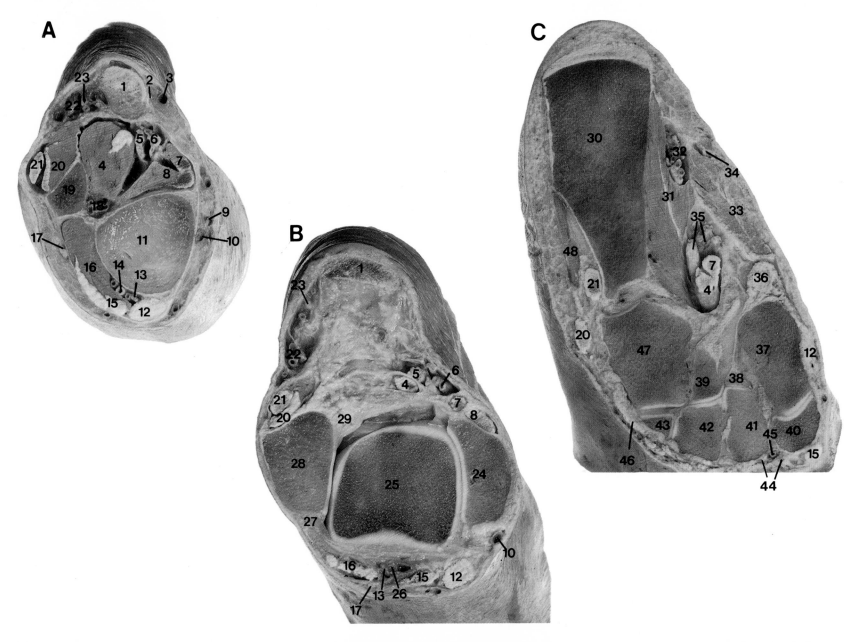

Sections of the foot

Sections of the right lower leg and foot

A Transverse, about 6 cm above the ankle joint
B Transverse, through the ankle joint
C Oblique, about 5 cm below the ankle joint

1 Tendo calcaneus
2 Plantaris
3 A tributary of great saphenous vein
4 Flexor hallucis longus
5 Tibial nerve
6 Posterior tibial vessels
7 Flexor digitorum longus
8 Tibialis posterior
9 Saphenous nerve
10 Great saphenous vein
11 Tibia
12 Tibialis anterior
13 Deep peroneal nerve
14 Anterior tibial vessels
15 Extensor hallucis longus
16 Extensor digitorum longus
17 Superficial peroneal nerve
18 Peroneal vessels
19 Fibula
20 Peroneus brevis
21 Peroneus longus
22 Small saphenous vein
23 Sural nerve
24 Medial malleolus

25 Talus
26 Dorsalis pedis artery
27 Anterior talofibular ligament
28 Lateral malleolus
29 Posterior talofibular ligament
30 Calcaneus
31 Flexor accessorius
32 Lateral plantar nerve and vessels
33 Abductor hallucis
34 Medial calcanean nerve
35 Medial plantar nerve and vessels
36 Tip of tuberosity of navicular and 8
37 Medial ⎤
38 Intermediate ⎬ cuneiform
39 Lateral ⎦
40 First ⎤
41 Second ⎬ metatarsal base
42 Third ⎥
43 Fourth ⎦
44 First dorsal interosseous
45 Deep plantar artery
46 Extensor digitorum brevis
47 Cuboid
48 Abductor digiti minimi

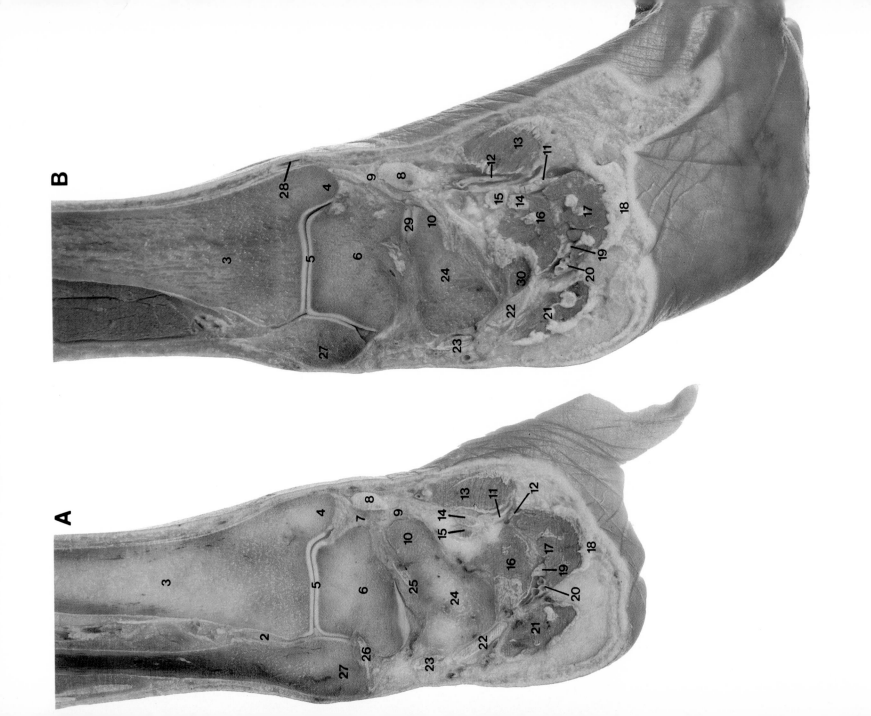

Sections of the foot

Coronal sections of the left ankle joint, in plantar flexion

A Through the posterior part of the talus, from behind

B About 1 cm in front of A, through the talocalcanean part of the talocalcaneonavicular joint, from behind

1 Fibula
2 Interosseous tibiofibular ligament
3 Tibia
4 Medial malleolus
5 Ankle joint
6 Talus
7 Deep part of medial (deltoid) ligament
8 Tibialis posterior
9 Medial ligament
10 Sustentaculum tali
11 Medial plantar nerve
12 Medial plantar artery
13 Abductor hallucis
14 Flexor digitorum longus
15 Flexor hallucis longus
16 Flexor accessorius
17 Flexor digitorum brevis
18 Plantar aponeurosis
19 Lateral plantar nerve
20 Lateral plantar vessels
21 Abductor digiti minimi
22 Peroneus longus
23 Peroneus brevis
24 Calcaneus
25 Interosseous talocalcanean ligament
26 Posterior talofibular ligament
27 Lateral malleolus
28 Great saphenous vein
29 Talocalcanean part of talocalcaneonavicular joint
30 Cuboid

● Joints, muscles and movements

At the ankle joint

Dorsiflexion: tibialis anterior, extensor hallucis longus, extensor digitorum longus, peroneus tertius.

Plantar flexion: gastrocnemius, soleus, plantaris, tibialis posterior, flexor hallucis longus, flexor digitorum longus.

At the talocalcanean and talocalcaneonavicular joints

Inversion: tibialis anterior and tibialis posterior.

Eversion: peroneus longus, peroneus brevis and peroneus tertius.

At the other small joints of the foot there are minor degrees of gliding or rotatory movements. At the transverse tarsal joint (page 33) a small amount of inversion and eversion occurs, but by far the greater part of these important movements takes place at the two joints beneath the talus. To visualise inversion and eversion, imagine the talus held firmly between the tibia and fibula, and the whole of the rest of the foot swivelling inwards or outwards underneath the talus. These movements do *not* take place at the ankle joint which essentially only allows dorsiflexion and plantar flexion.

The actions of muscles on the toes are indicated by their names but the part played by the interossei and lumbricals requires some explanation (apart from the abduction and adduction produced by the interossei and referred to on page 67). Briefly the interossei and lumbricals work together to flex the metatarsophalangeal joints and extend the interphalangeal joints; these apparently contradictory actions on different joints by the same muscles can be explained as follows.

The interossei (both plantar and dorsal) are attached mainly to the sides of the proximal phalanges but also into the dorsal digital expansions; the lumbricals are usually attached entirely to the expansions. Because of the position of these attachments in relation to the axis of movement of the metatarsophalangeal joints, the interossei and lumbricals plantar flex these joints.

Because the lumbrical attachments and parts of the interosseous attachments are to the basal angles of the expansions, the line of pull is transmitted to the dorsal surfaces of the toes distal to the metatarsophalangeal joints, and so the interphalangeal joints are extended.

In most feet the interosseous attachment to the expansions is minimal, and it is the lumbricals that are mainly responsible for assisting the long and short extensor tendons in extending the toes, keeping them straight and stabilised against the pull of the flexors which tend to make them buckle, especially during the push-off phase of walking when flexor hallucis longus and flexor digitorum longus are contracting strongly.

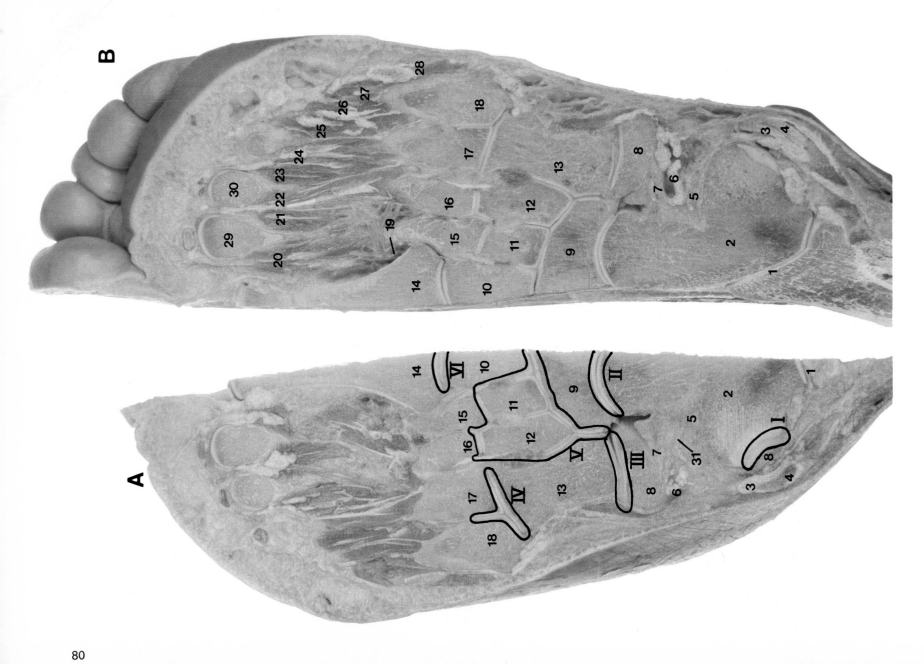

Sections of the foot

Oblique horizontal sections through the left foot

(The plane of section is shown in the small scale illustration. The surfaces A and B have been separated and are viewed as pages in an opened book. For an explanation of the joint cavities outlined in A see the note below.)

1 Ankle joint
2 Talus
3 Peroneus brevis
4 Peroneus longus
5 Interosseous talocalcanean ligament
6 Extensor digitorum brevis
7 Cervical ligament
8 Calcaneus
9 Navicular
10 Medial ⎤
11 Intermediate ⎬ cuneiform
12 Lateral ⎦
13 Cuboid
14 First ⎤
15 Second ⎥
16 Third ⎬ metatarsal base
17 Fourth ⎥
18 Fifth ⎦
19 Deep plantar branch of first dorsal metatarsal artery
20 First dorsal ⎤
21 Second dorsal ⎥
22 First plantar ⎥
23 Third dorsal ⎬ interosseous
24 Second plantar ⎥
25 Fourth dorsal ⎥
26 Third plantar ⎦
27 Flexor digiti minimi brevis
28 Abductor digiti minimi
29 Head of second metatarsal
30 Head of third metatarsal
31 Inferior extensor retinaculum

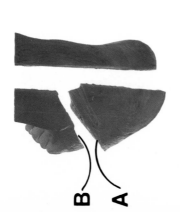

● The cavities of a number of synovial joints in the foot are continuous with one another to the extent that there are normally six synovial cavities associated with the tarsal bones:

I   The talocalcanean joint cavity.
II   The talocalcaneonavicular joint cavity.
III The calcaneocuboid joint cavity.
IV   The cuboideometatarsal joint cavity (between the cuboid and the bases of the fourth and fifth metatarsals).
V   The cuneonavicular and cuneometatarsal joint cavity (between the navicular, the three cuneiforms and the bases of the second, third and fourth metatarsals).
VI   The medial cuneometatarsal joint cavity (between the medial cuneiform and the base of the first metatarsal).

Parts of all the above cavities can be seen in the foot sectioned here; they are indicated by the black lines in A and numbered as above. (The cuboideonavicular joint is usually a fibrous union but in this specimen it is synovial and continuous with the cuneonavicular joint cavity.)

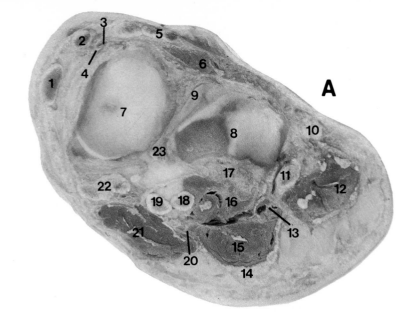

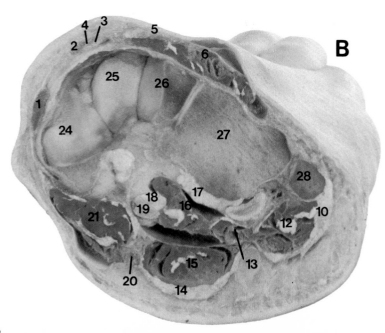

Sections of the foot

Sections of the right tarsus (looking from the heel towards the toes)

A Through the transverse tarsal joint, proximal to the navicular
B Through the cuneonavicular joint, distal to the navicular

1 Tibialis anterior
2 Extensor hallucis longus
3 Dorsalis pedis artery
4 Deep peroneal nerve
5 Extensor digitorum longus
6 Extensor digitorum brevis
7 Posterior articular surface of navicular (for talus)
8 Posterior articular surface of cuboid (for calcaneus)
9 Anterior tip of calcaneus
10 Peroneus brevis
11 Peroneus longus
12 Abductor digiti minimi
13 Lateral plantar nerve and vessels
14 Plantar aponeurosis
15 Flexor digitorum brevis
16 Flexor accessorius
17 Plantar calcaneocuboid (short plantar) ligament
18 Flexor hallucis longus
19 Flexor digitorum longus
20 Medial plantar nerve and vessels
21 Abductor hallucis
22 Tibialis posterior
23 Plantar calcaneonavicular (spring) ligament
24 Medial ⎤
25 Intermediate ⎬ cuneiform
26 Lateral ⎦
27 Cuboid
28 Tuberosity of fifth metatarsal

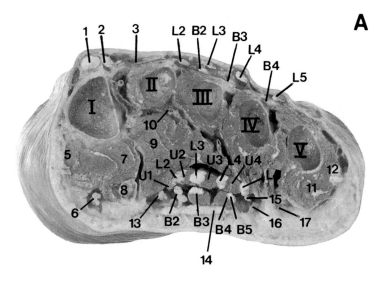

A

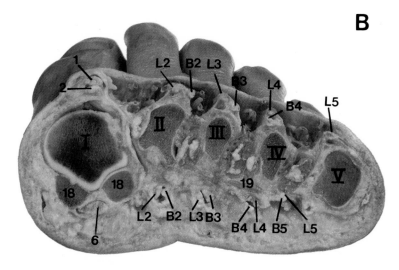

B

Sections of the foot

Sections of the right metatarsus (looking from the heel towards the toes)

   A Through the metatarsal shafts

   B Through the heads of the first and fifth metatarsals (about 2.5 cm distal to A).

      (On the dorsum the tendons of extensor digitorum longus to the appropriate toes are numbered L2–L5 and those of extensor digitorum brevis B2–B4. Similarly in the sole flexor digitorum longus tendons are numbered L2–L5 and flexor digitorum brevis B2–B5, with the lumbrical muscles U1–U4. The metatarsals are numbered in Roman figures.)

  1 Extensor hallucis longus
  2 Extensor hallucis brevis
  3 Arcuate artery
  4 Deep plantar artery
  5 Abductor hallucis
  6 Proper plantar digital nerve of great toe
  7 Flexor hallucis brevis
  8 Flexor hallucis longus
  9 Oblique head of adductor hallucis
10 Second plantar metatarsal artery
11 Flexor digiti minimi brevis
12 Abductor digiti minimi
13 Common plantar digital branches of medial plantar nerve
14 Plantar aponeurosis
15 Deep branch of lateral plantar nerve
16 Fourth common plantar digital nerve
17 Proper plantar digital nerve of fifth toe
18 Sesamoid bone
19 Transverse head of adductor hallucis

The great toe

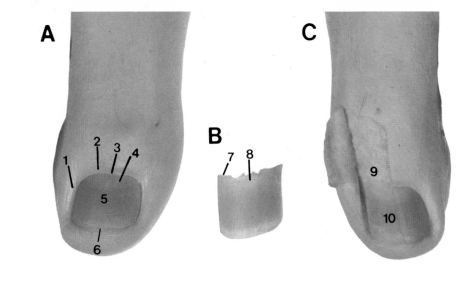

The dorsum, nail, and sections of the great toe

A Dorsum of the right great toe
B Nail
C Nail bed of the left great toe
D Sagittal section of the right great toe, from the lateral side
E Coronal section of the distal phalanx of the right great toe

1 Nail wall
2 Nail fold
3 Eponychium
4 Lunule
5 Body
6 Free border ⎤ of nail
7 Occult border ⎥
8 Root ⎦
9 Germinal matrix ⎤ of nail bed
10 Sterile matrix ⎦
11 Head of first metatarsal
12 Capsule of metatarsophalangeal joint
13 Attachment of extensor hallucis brevis
14 Proximal phalanx
15 Capsule of interphalangeal joint
16 Attachment of extensor hallucis longus
17 Distal phalanx
18 Septa of pulp space
19 Attachment of flexor hallucis longus
20 Plantar ligament of interphalangeal joint
21 Flexor hallucis longus
22 Sesamoid bone

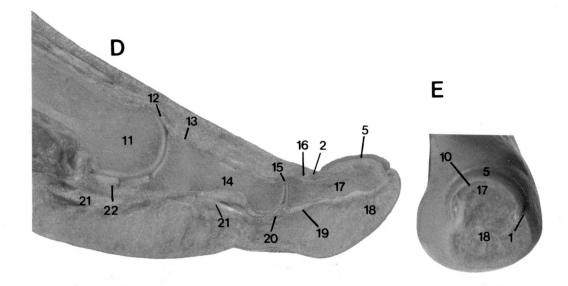

Radiography of the foot

Anteroposterior and lateral radiographs

A Anteroposterior view, weight-bearing

B Lateral view, weight-bearing

1 Calcaneus
2 Head of talus
3 Navicular
4 Cuboid
5 Medial ⎫
6 Intermediate ⎬ cuneiform
7 Lateral ⎭
8 Second metatarsal
9 Sesamoid bone
10 Proximal ⎫ phalanx
11 Middle ⎬ of second
12 Distal ⎭ toe
13 Ankle joint
14 Talocalcanean joint
15 Calcaneocuboid joint
16 Talonavicular part of
   talocalcaneonavicular joint

● In A. note the shadow of the great toe nail.

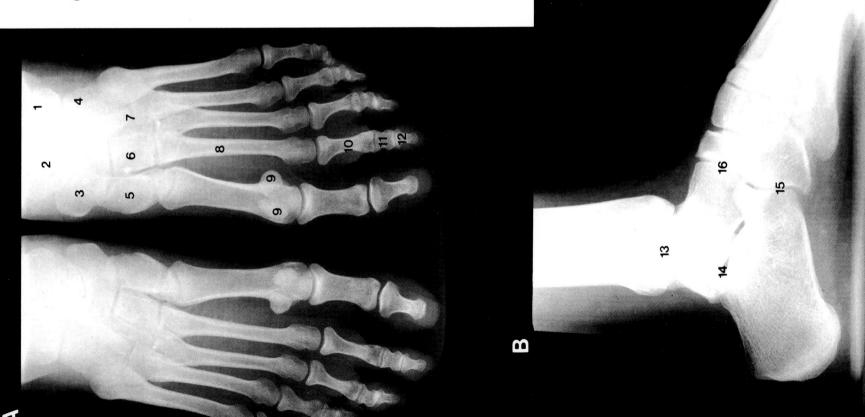

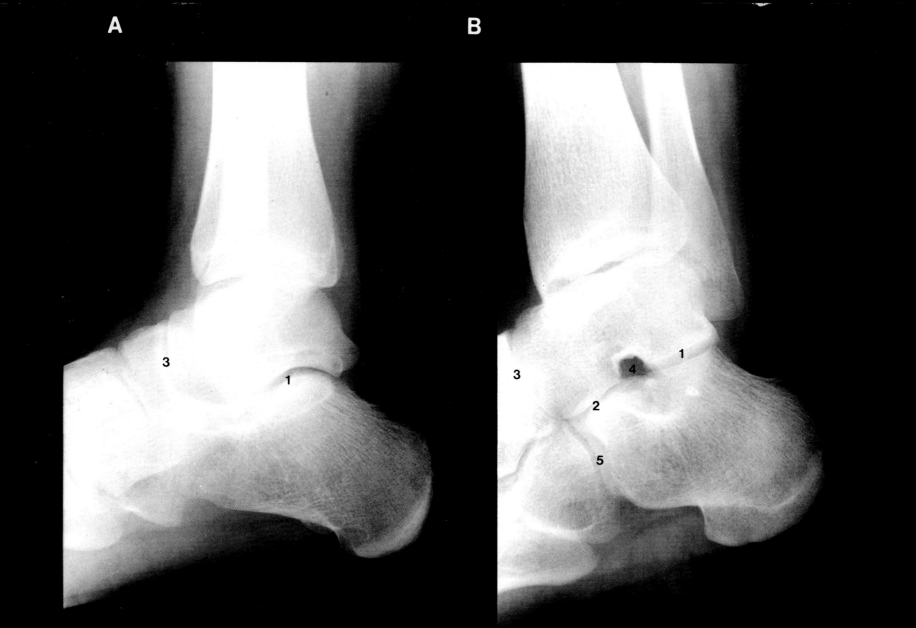

Radiography of the foot

Miscellaneous radiographs

A Lateral view to show
  talocalcanean joint
B Oblique lateral view to
  show tarsal sinus
C View standing on tip-toe
D View to show sesamoid bones

1 Talocalcanean joint
2 Talocalcanean part*
3 Talonavicular part*
4 Tarsal sinus
5 Calcaneocuboid joint

*of talocalcaneonavicular joint

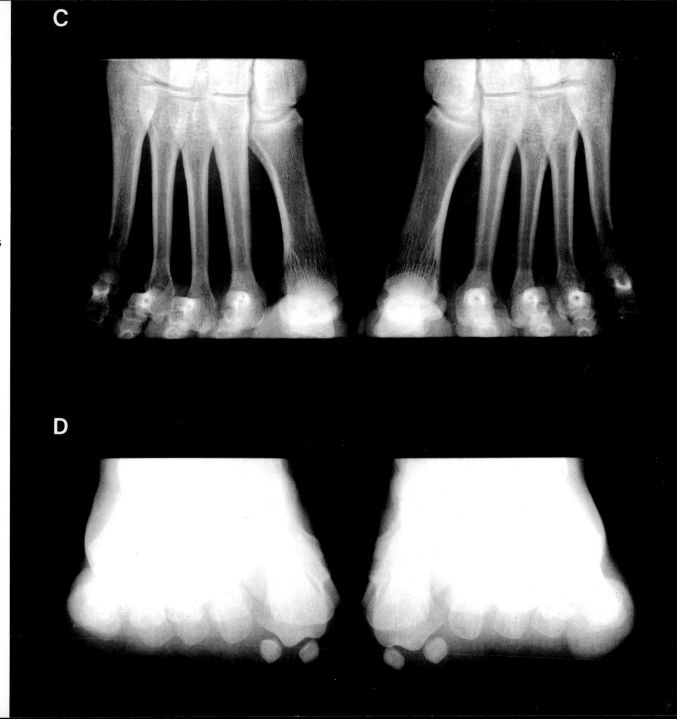

Appendix
Muscles

Extensor muscles of the front of the leg and dorsum of the foot

Tibialis anterior
From the upper two-thirds of the lateral surface of the tibia and the adjoining part of the interosseous membrane.
To the medial surface of the medial cuneiform and base of the first metatarsal.
Deep peroneal nerve, L4 and 5.
Dorsiflexion and inversion of the foot.

Extensor hallucis longus
From the middle third of the medial surface of the fibula.
To the base of the distal phalanx of the great toe.
Deep peroneal nerve, L5 and S1.
Extension of the great toe and dorsiflexion of the foot.

Extensor digitorum longus
From the upper two-thirds of the medial surface of the fibula.
To the four lateral toes by a tendon to each, attached to the middle and distal phalanges.
Deep peroneal nerve, L5 and S1.
Extension of the four lateral toes and dorsiflexion of the foot.

Peroneus tertius
From the lower third of the medial surface of the fibula as a continuation of extensor digitorum longus.
To the base of the fifth metatarsal.
Deep peroneal nerve, L5 and S1.
Dorsiflexion and eversion of the foot.

Peroneal muscles of the lateral side of the leg

Peroneus longus
From the upper two-thirds of the lateral surface of the fibula.
To the lateral side of the medial cuneiform and base of the first metatarsal.
Superficial peroneal nerve, L5, S1 and 2.
Plantar flexion and eversion of the foot.

Peroneus brevis
From the lower two-thirds of the lateral surface of the fibula.
To the tuberosity of the base of the fifth metatarsal.
Superficial peroneal nerve, L5, S1 and 2.
Plantar flexion and eversion of the foot.

Flexor muscles of the back of the leg and sole of the foot

Gastrocnemius
Medial head from the upper posterior part of the medial condyle of the femur, and the lateral head from the lateral surface of the lateral condyle of the femur.
To the middle of the posterior surface of the calcaneus by the tendo calcaneus (in association with soleus).
Tibial nerve, S1 and 2.
Plantar flexion of the foot (and flexion of the knee).

Soleus
From the soleal line and upper part of the medial border of tibia, a tendinous arch over the popliteal vessels and tibial nerve, and the upper part of the posterior surface of the fibula.
To the middle of the posterior surface of the calcaneus by the tendo calcaneus (in association with gastrocnemius).
Tibial nerve, S1 and 2.
Plantar flexion of the foot.

Plantaris
From the lateral supracondylar line of the femur.
To the medial side of the tendo calcaneus.
Tibial nerve, S1 and 2.
Plantar flexion of the foot (and flexion of the knee).

Tibialis posterior
From the posterior surface of the interosseus membrane and adjacent posterior surfaces of the tibia and fibula.
To the tuberosity of the navicular, with slips to other tarsal bones (except the talus) and the middle three metatarsals.
Tibial nerve, L4 and 5.
Plantar flexion and inversion of the foot.

Flexor hallucis longus
From the lower two-thirds of the posterior surface of the fibula.
To the plantar surface of the base of the distal phalanx of the great toe.
Tibial nerve, S2 and 3.
Plantar flexion of the great toe and foot.

Flexor digitorum longus
From the medial part of the posterior surface of the tibia below the soleal line.
To the four lateral toes by a tendon to each, attached to the plantar surface of the base of the distal phalanx.
Tibial nerve, S2 and 3.
Plantar flexion of the four lateral toes and foot.

Muscles of the sole of the foot

First layer

Abductor hallucis

From the medial process of the calcanean tuberosity and the plantar aponeurosis.

To the medial side of the proximal phalanx of the great toe.

Medial plantar nerve, S2 and 3.

Abduction and plantar flexion of the great toe.

Flexor digitorum brevis

From the medial process of the calcanean tuberosity and the deep surface of the central part of the plantar aponeurosis.

To the four lateral toes by a tendon to each; the tendon divides into two slips (to allow the flexor digitorum longus tendon to pass between them) which are attached to the sides of the middle phalanx.

Medial plantar nerve, S2 and 3.

Plantar flexion of the four lateral toes.

Abductor digiti minimi

From the lateral and medial processes of the calcanean tuberosity and the plantar aponeurosis.

To the lateral side of the base of the proximal phalanx of the fifth toe (with flexor digiti minimi brevis).

Lateral plantar nerve, S2 and 3.

Abduction and plantar flexion of the fifth toe.

Second layer

Flexor accessorius (quadratus plantae)

From the (concave) medial surface of the calcaneus and from the plantar surface of the calcaneus in front of the lateral process of the tuberosity.

To the lateral border of flexor digitorum longus before the division into four tendons.

Lateral plantar nerve, S2 and 3.

Assistance with plantar flexion of the four lateral toes.

Lumbricals

First lumbrical from the medial border of the first tendon of flexor digitorum longus.

Second, third and fourth lumbricals from the four adjoining tendons of flexor digitorum longus.

To the medial sides of the dorsal digital expansions of the tendons of extensor digitorum longus.

First lumbrical – medial plantar nerve; second, third and fourth lumbrical by the lateral plantar nerve, S2 and 3.

Plantar flexion at the four lateral metatarsophalangeal joints and extension at interphalangeal joints.

Third layer

Flexor hallucis brevis

From the plantar surface of the cuboid and lateral cuneiform.

By a tendon to each side of the base of the proximal phalanx of the great toe, the medial tendon joining with that of abductor hallucis and the lateral with adductor hallucis; there is a sesamoid bone in each tendon.

Medial plantar nerve, S2 and 3.

Plantar flexion of the metatarsophalangeal joint of the great toe.

Adductor hallucis

Oblique head from the bases of the second, third and fourth metatarsals.

Transverse head from the plantar metatarsophalangeal ligaments of the third, fourth and fifth toes.

To the lateral side of the base of the proximal phalanx of the great toe, with part of flexor hallucis brevis.

Lateral plantar nerve, S2 and 3.

Adduction of the great toe.

Flexor digiti minimi brevis

From the plantar surface of the base of the first metatarsal.

To the lateral side of the base of proximal phalanx of the fifth toe, with abductor digiti minimi.

Lateral plantar nerve, S2 and 3.

Plantar flexion of the metatarsophalangeal joint of the fifth toe.

Fourth layer

Dorsal interossei (four)

From adjacent sides of the bodies of a pair of metatarsals.

To the bases of proximal phalanges and the dorsal digital expansions. First and second to the medial and lateral sides of the second toe; third and fourth to the lateral sides of the third and fourth toes.

Lateral plantar nerve, S2 and 3.

Plantar flexion of the metatarsophalangeal joints and extension (dorsiflexion) of the interphalangeal joints of the second, third and fourth toes; abduction of the same toes.

Plantar interossei (three)

From the bases and medial sides of the third, fourth and fifth metatarsals.

To the medial sides of the bases of the proximal phalanges and dorsal digital expansions of the corresponding toes.

Lateral plantar nerve, S2 and 3.

Plantar flexion of the metatarsophalangeal joints and extension (dorsiflexion) of the interphalangeal joints of the third, fourth and fifth toes; adduction of the same toes.

Nerves

Branches of the medial plantar nerve
Trunk, giving off
Nerve to abductor hallucis
Nerve to flexor digitorum brevis
Proper plantar digital nerve of great toe, giving off
Nerve to flexor hallucis brevis
First common plantar digital nerve, giving off
Nerve to first lumbrical
Proper plantar digital nerves of first cleft
Second common plantar digital nerve, giving off
Proper plantar digital nerves of second cleft
Third common plantar digital nerve, giving off
Proper plantar digital nerves of third cleft.

Branches of the lateral plantar nerve
Trunk, giving off
Nerve to flexor accessorius
Nerve to abductor digiti minimi
Superficial branch, giving off
Fourth common plantar digital nerve, giving off
Proper plantar digital nerves of fourth cleft
Proper plantar digital nerve of fifth toe, giving off
Nerve to flexor digiti minimi brevis
Nerve to third plantar interosseous
Nerve to fourth dorsal interosseous
Deep branch, giving off
Nerve to adductor hallucis
Nerves to second, third and fourth lumbricals
Nerves to first, second and third dorsal interossei
Nerves to first and second plantar interossei.

Arteries

Branches of the dorsalis pedis artery
Lateral tarsal
Medial tarsal
First dorsal metatarsal, giving off
Deep plantar (perforating) branch, to complete plantar arch
Dorsal digital branch to medial side of great toe
Dorsal digital branches to first cleft
Arcuate, giving off
Second dorsal metatarsal, giving off
Perforating branches
Dorsal digital branches to second cleft
Third dorsal metatarsal, giving off
Perforating branches
Dorsal digital branches to third cleft
Fourth dorsal metatarsal, giving off
Perforating branches
Dorsal digital branches to fourth cleft
Dorsal digital branch to lateral side of fifth toe.

Branches of the lateral plantar artery

    Plantar arch, giving off
        First plantar metatarsal, giving off
            Plantar digital artery to medial side of great toe
            Plantar digital arteries to first cleft
        Second, third and fourth plantar metatarsal arteries, each
            giving off
            Plantar digital arteries to second, third and fourth clefts
                respectively
        Perforating branches
    Plantar digital artery to lateral side of fifth toe.

Branches of the medial plantar artery

    Anastomotic branch to plantar digital artery of medial side of the
        great toe
    Superficial digital branches to anastomose with first, second and
        third plantar metatarsal arteries.

Index

Abduction 21, 79
Acetabulum 10–13
Adduction 21, 79
Ankle 11, 43, 50, 54
– joint 11, 16, 27, 38, 61, 62, 68, 73–80, 85
Aponeurosis, plantar 33, 55, 63, 64, 73, 74, 78, 82, 83
Arch, dorsal venous 20, 50, 52, 53
– lateral longitudinal 32, 33
– medial longitudinal 31–33
– plantar 61, 65–67, 74
– posterior (vein) 51, 52
– transverse 33
Artery, arteries, see also Vessels
– anterior tibial 52, 55, 61
– arcuate 60, 61, 83
– deep plantar 60, 61, 76, 80, 83
– dorsal digital 60, 61
– dorsal metatarsal 60, 61, 67, 80
– dorsalis pedis 20, 23, 56, 60–62, 76, 82
– lateral plantar 61, 64–67
– medial plantar 64–67, 78
– perforating 60, 61, 67
– peroneal 60, 61
– plantar arch 61, 65–67, 74
– plantar digital 61, 67
– plantar metatarsal 64–67, 83
– popliteal 18
– posterior tibial 20–23, 57, 58, 67
– superficial digital 64, 67
– tarsal 61
Astragalus 25

B

Base of metatarsal 20, 27, 30, 68, 71
– of phalanx 27, 30
Body of femur 10–16
– of fibula 10, 12, 16

– of long bone 11
– of metatarsal 27, 30
– of nail 84
– of phalanx 27, 30
– of talus 34, 36
– weight 31
Bones, see also individual names
– of foot 24–49
– of lower limb 10–16
Bursa 28, 44, 48, 49, 62, 73, 74
Buttock 11, 12

C

Calcaneum 27
Calcaneus 20–27, 30–32, 44, 51, 55, 57–59, 62, 63, 68, 73–82, 85
Calf of leg 52
Capsule of ankle joint 38, 42
– of interphalangeal joint 84
– of metatarsophalangeal joint 68, 70, 84
– of talocalcanean joint 45
– of talocalcaneonavicular joint 38, 42, 45, 68
Cartilage 27
– of plantar calcaneonavicular ligament 62
Cleft of toes 50, 61, 63, 66, 67
Condyles of femur 10–16
– of tibia 10–16
Cuboid bone 24, 26, 30, 46, 49, 74–82, 85
Cuneiform bones 24, 26, 30, 32, 47, 72–74, 76, 80, 82, 85

D

Dermatome 50, 63
Digits 25
Dissections 50–84
Dorsiflexion 21, 22, 79
Dorsum of foot 19, 20, 25, 50, 54, 56, 60, 67
– of great toe 84

E

Epicondyles of femur 16
Eponychium 84
Eversion 20, 21, 79
Expansion, dorsal digital 56, 59, 60, 79
Extension 22, 79

F

Fascia 19, 50–54

Femur 10–16
Fibula 10, 12, 16, 25, 27, 36–42, 55, 56, 59, 60, 62, 65, 75–78
Flat foot 31
Flexion 21, 22
Foot 10–16
– arches 32, 33
– arteries 61, 67
– bones 24–49
– joints 33, 62, 79
– ligaments 68–71
– movements 21, 31, 33, 79
– muscles of dorsum 19
– – of sole 64–67
– nerves 50, 63
Forearm 31
Fossa, malleolar 36
– popliteal 12, 52

G

Girdle, pelvic 11
Gluteal region 11
Groove for flexor hallucis longus 34, 36, 44, 69, 71
– for peroneus brevis 36
– for peroneus longus 46, 69
– for sesamoid bones 48
– for tibialis posterior 36, 69

H

Hallux 25
Hamstrings 12–14
Hand 31
Head(s) of adductor hallucis 66, 74, 83
– of femur 10, 12, 16
– of fibula 10, 12, 16
– of gastrocnemius 12
– of metatarsals 20, 22, 27, 30, 31, 80, 83, 84
– of talus 34, 36, 40, 62, 68, 85
Heel 25, 27, 31, 50, 51
Hip 11
– bone 10, 11, 14, 16
– joint 11, 16

I

Iliac crest 10, 12, 16
Ilium 10, 12
Imprint of foot 21, 31
Inversion 20, 21, 79
Ischium 10, 12

J

Joint(s) 32, 79
– ankle 11, 16, 27, 38, 61, 62, 68, 73–80, 85
– calcaneocuboid 32, 68, 75, 80, 85, 86
– cavities of foot 80, 81
– cuboideometatarsal 32, 75, 80
– cuboideonavicular 32
– cuneocuboid 32
– cuneometatarsal 32, 73, 80
– cuneonavicular 32, 73, 80, 82
– hip 11, 16
– inferior tibiofibular 11, 16
– intercuneiform 32
– intermetatarsal 32
– interphalangeal 32
– knee 11, 16
– metatarsophalangeal 32, 50, 56, 68, 70, 71, 73, 75, 79, 84
– midtarsal 33
– movements 79
– pubic symphysis 11
– sacro-iliac 11
– subtalar 62
– superior tibiofibular 11, 16
– talocalcanean 32, 62, 73–75, 79, 80, 85, 86
– talocalcaneonavicular 32, 38, 62, 68, 73, 74, 78–80, 85, 86
– talocrural 62
– tarsometatarsal 32
– transverse tarsal 33, 79, 82

K

Knee 11
– joint 11, 16

L

Layers of plantar aponeurosis 63
– of muscles of sole 64–67
Leg 11, 18, 19, 76
Ligament(s) 28, 68–71
– anterior talofibular 38, 42, 60, 68, 76
– anterior tibiofibular 38, 42, 68
– bifurcate 28, 45, 68
– calcaneofibular 38, 42, 44, 68
– cervical 45, 62, 68, 80
– collateral 68, 70
– deep transverse metatarsal 71
– deltoid 38, 42, 45, 62, 68–70, 78
– dorsal calcaneocuboid 68
– dorsal cuneonavicular 68

– dorsal metatarsal 68
– dorsal tarsometatarsal 68, 70
– inguinal 10
– interosseous talocalcanean 45, 62, 73, 74, 78, 80
– interosseous tibiofibular 36, 38, 78
– lateral talocalcanean 45
– long plantar 28, 33, 68–71
– medial (of ankle) 38, 42, 45, 62, 68–70, 78
– medial talocalcanean 45
– patellar 10, 18
– plantar calcaneocuboid 28, 33, 71, 82
– plantar calcaneonavicular 28, 33, 34, 62, 71–74, 82
– plantar cuneonavicular 71
– plantar of interphalangeal joint 84
– plantar of metatarsophalangeal joint 71
– plantar tarsometatarsal 71
– posterior talofibular 38, 69, 76, 78
– posterior tibiofibular 38, 42, 69
– short plantar 28, 33, 71
– spring 28, 33, 34, 62, 71–74, 82
– superficial transverse metatarsal 63, 64
– talonavicular 70
Lower limb 10–16
Lunule 84
Lymph nodes and vessels 10, 52

M

Malleolus, lateral 10, 12, 16, 20–23, 36, 50–60, 68, 69, 76, 78
– medial 10–14, 20–23, 36, 40, 50–58, 68–70, 76, 78
Matrix of nail 84
Membrane, interosseous 38, 52, 60, 69
Metatarsal bones 20–26, 30–32, 48, 49, 67–76, 80–85
Metatarsus 25, 83
Movements, definition 21
– joint 79
Muscle(s) 19, 79
– abductor digiti minimi 28, 53, 54, 60, 63–67, 73–83
– abductor hallucis 28, 52, 55, 58, 63–67, 72, 76, 78, 82, 83
– adductor hallucis 28, 64–66, 74, 83
– attachments to bones 28, 38, 42, 45
– biceps femoris 12, 13, 16, 18
– dorsal interosseous 28, 56, 60, 61, 64–67, 76, 79, 80
– extensor digitorum brevis 18–22, 28, 45, 53–56, 59–62, 74–76, 80–83
– extensor digitorum longus 10, 16–23, 28, 50, 54–56, 59–62, 74, 76, 79, 82, 83
– extensor hallucis brevis 28, 56, 72, 83, 84
– extensor hallucis longus 10, 18–23, 54–56, 58–62, 68, 70–74, 76, 79, 82–84
– flexor accessorius 28, 29, 64–67, 73, 74, 76, 78, 82
– flexor digiti minimi brevis 28, 64–67, 75, 80, 83
– flexor digitorum brevis 28, 33, 63–67, 71, 74, 82, 83

– flexor digitorum longus 14, 18–22, 28, 33, 57, 58, 62, 64–67, 71–74, 76–79, 82, 83
– flexor hallucis brevis 27, 28, 63–66, 83
– flexor hallucis longus 18–22, 28, 33, 36, 38, 44, 57, 58, 62, 64–74, 76, 78, 79, 82–84
– of foot 18, 19, 28, 50–67
– of forearm and hand 31
– gastrocnemius 10–19, 79
– gluteus maximus 12, 16
– gluteus medius 16
– gracilis 10, 14, 18
– hamstring 12–14
– of leg 18, 19
– of lower limb 10–16
– lumbrical 56, 63–65, 74, 79, 83
– opponens digiti minimi 28
– peroneus brevis 18–22, 28, 36, 54–57, 59–62, 75–82
– peroneus longus 16–22, 27, 28, 33, 46, 47, 53, 54, 57, 59–62, 67, 69, 71–82
– peroneus tertius 18, 19, 28, 38, 55, 56, 59, 79
– plantar interosseous 28, 64–67, 80
– plantaris 18, 19, 28, 57, 58, 76, 79
– popliteus 18, 19
– quadratus plantae 29
– quadriceps 10
– rectus femoris 10
– sartorius 10, 14, 18
– semimembranosus 12–14, 18
– semitendinosus 12–14, 18
– of sole 19, 64–67
– soleus 10–19, 57–59, 79
– tensor fasciae latae 10, 16
– tibialis anterior 10, 16–22, 27, 28, 33, 47, 50, 54–62, 66, 67, 70–74, 76, 79, 82
– tibialis posterior 10, 16–22, 28, 33, 36, 56–58, 62, 67, 69–74, 76–79, 82
– of upper limb 31
– vastus lateralis 10, 16
– vastus medialis 10, 14

N

Nail 84, 85
Navicular bone 20–26, 30, 32, 46, 62, 66, 67, 70–74, 76, 80, 82, 85
Neck of femur 10, 12, 16
– of fibula 10, 12, 16
– of talus 34, 40
Nerve(s) to abductor digiti minimi 65
– to abductor hallucis 66
– to adductor hallucis 66
– common peroneal 12, 16, 18
– cutaneous 50, 63
– deep peroneal 50, 55, 60, 62, 76, 82
– dorsal digital 50, 52